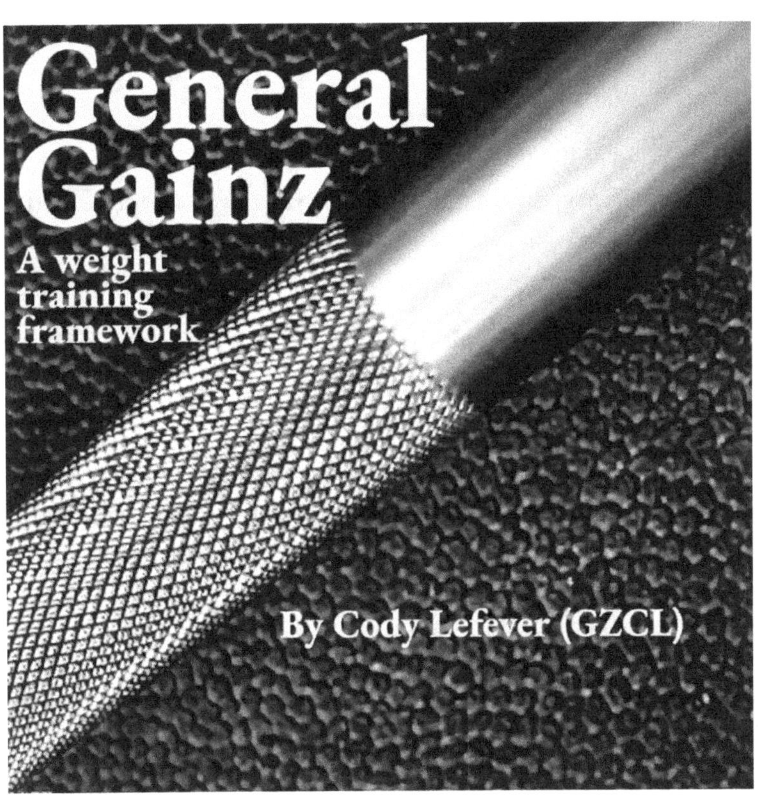
General
Gainz
A weight
training
framework
By Cody Lefever (GZCL)

ISBN: 978-1-7351202-5-6

Printed in the United States of America

First Edition

For permissions, inquiries, or more information, contact:

www.gainzfever.com

A special thanks to my wife for supporting me while I spent countless hours in the gym. You are my rock that I happily lift. I love you.

Another heartfelt thanks to Benjamin Kühne, who helped edit this book and who, as a client of mine, helped me explore several progressions within the General Gainz framework.

To all my clients and gym members, thank you for your support and encouragement. I would not be where I am without you either.

And to all my readers, thank you for your time and your sweat. I pray you receive an abundance of size, strength, and endurance.

Glory to God in the highest.

Contents

Results

General Gainz has led to thousands of pounds in personal records for both me and those who have followed my training methods online. While developing GG, I reached my all-time heaviest bodyweight and set PRs across multiple lifts while training daily. You don't have to train every day with GG, but I chose to, and I believe it improved my results. With GG, I grew bigger, stronger, and fitter than I was when I competed at the national and world levels in powerlifting.

At my peak as a powerlifter, I squatted 523 pounds. Nearly a decade later, using GG instead of a traditional powerlifting approach, I reached 525. Not much of a 1RM improvement, but context is important: I wasn't training for a one rep max. During the same period, I also hit personal records for high-rep squats, including 135 lbs. for 102 reps, 185 for 76, 225 for 51, 275 for 37, and 315 for 26. While I value my 1RM personal records set using GG, I've come to prefer higher-rep training as I age.

Other PRs I set during this period are a 3RM squat of 500 lbs., a 3RM press of 225 lbs. with a 1RM max of 250 lbs., a 3RM beltless deadlift of 585 lbs. with a 1RM of 600 lbs. (also beltless). These were completed around 200 lbs. in bodyweight.

GG shifted my training from a percentage-based approach to one focused on day-to-day rep ability, with more consistent volume and intensity regulation. This allowed me to train frequently, stay injury-free, and continue setting lifetime PRs a decade after my previous bests, all without hormone therapy or performance-enhancing substances.

My clients, including national- and world-level competitors, have achieved similar success. Since I first shared GG's structure online, others have refined and expanded it, proving its effectiveness. Search GZCL and General Gainz, and you'll find years of results from lifters who have used these principles successfully. General Gainz works.

For an awe-inspiring result, read this excellent guest post on my blog: Swole at Every Height: 365 Days and Counting, written by a client of mine who used General Gainz to build impressive size, strength, and stamina.

What is General Gainz?

General Gainz (GG) is a flexible weight-training framework suitable for both new and experienced lifters, from which specific training plans can be created. This guide describes the concept and theory of GG. Later sections provide examples and specific applications to inspire the training plans you develop, deepening your understanding of GG.

What makes GG unique is its use of Volume Drop Sets (VDS), which set it apart from other popular weight-training approaches. A volume drop set is a higher-rep set followed by lower-rep sets, all with the same weight.

Example: 10 Rep Max (10RM) followed by additional sets of 5 reps each, using the same weight.

This is the snowflake atop the General Gainz iceberg; the surface of something much more vast and expansive.

Volume Drop Sets limit fatigue while allowing you to maintain high rep quality, such as positioning and bar speed. These factors will enable you to "master a weight," as I call it. When a weight is mastered, you can lift it for more reps and more often, indicating it has become easier and you have gotten stronger. This can be done without forcing weight increases from workout to workout, often resulting in grinding reps and lifters grinding themselves out of the gym entirely.

Volume Drop Sets also limit the change in weight between sets as rep quality declines due to fatigue accumulation. This results in less time spent calculating loads and shuffling plates, leaving more time to train. The idea is that you have an RM target and after completing that priority set, you keep lifting the same weight for more sets of lower reps; this is practice and capacity building, the means of mastering weights.

General Gainz provides many options for progression. These I later describe. But GG is vast. So not everything is provided. Nor could it be. I have pushed the boundaries and peeled back many layers. Still, I am often introduced to innovative ideas developed by others using this framework for their training, either through my coaching or by learning about others' use of GG on social media, where I first began discussing it more than seven years ago.

General Gainz provides specific actions and sets limits based on your results from one workout to the next. Plateaus are short-lived because the next step is an inherent consequence of the previous one. Outcomes inform progression, not hypothetical calculations. What actions to take in your next workout is never a mystery. Because of its intuitive progression options, progress is steady with GG (as long as you remain consistent with your gym effort and patient with the process).

Determine your progression route and move forward. Let results inform your next step, and the one after. You will achieve feats once thought unreachable by taking ownership of your progress with GG. When you own your progress, you get more of it.

Reasoned experimentation is advised. That is how GG came about, after all. I can only report my experience and relay others', so train accordingly. Fold your training experience into this progression concept, thereby expanding it as it develops you, as has been my experience, and that of many.

I've spent seven years developing this framework. Multitudes have contributed to the exploration of this vast training system, aiding GG's development. You will also find a novel use of GG. The effort, theirs and yours, is appreciated.

The Training Feedback Loop

Training with GG isn't about "trusting the process." Instead, it provides clear metrics to understand how your actions affect results. What you do produces either positive or negative outcomes; those outcomes guide your next steps. Over time, you'll improve your decision-making in the gym, leading to better progress.

Always record your training data. This feedback is crucial for refining future workouts and improving efficiency. But not all data is useful. Focus on the information that matters most for your current phase and goals.

For example, during a high-volume phase, rest times may matter less than in a strength-focused phase; the data's value is goal dependent and therefore an aspect of individualization—don't emphasize all data equally, you'll drown in useless information that mystifies rather than clarifies.

But many oversimplify progress by thinking that training hard is the key to success. They push harder until progress stops, then either deload (training too easy) or try even harder (which calls into question whether they were training hard at all before). This can work temporarily, but often leads to burnout, fatigue, and quitting.

The long-term solution isn't a simple "train harder or easier" mindset. It is about understanding the variables that affect your training and adjusting them to ensure consistent progress. Think of your training as a machine where your actions and outcomes drive momentum. Instead of pushing to extremes, adjust variables to maintain a balanced effort. Over time, you'll discover what works best for you in a machine that has taken you far.

In short, train smart by using your data to guide decisions. Adapt where needed and avoid getting bogged down in unnecessary details. As you train, you'll learn what data is truly valuable and how to use it to progress.

From General to Specific

The "general" in General Gainz refers to the framework's nature: it is a general framework from which specific progressions and workouts can be derived, making your goals achievable.

Example workouts and progression models are provided in the final sections of this guide. Consider them templates for general scenarios, though they still lack genuine specificity. Make them your own and take charge of your training by substituting exercises and letting your performance in today's session dictate how you progress in the next.

Your creativity, initiative, and effort will fill that gap in specificity.

Variety & Specificity

Variety and specificity are key when using a GG-based training plan, and they should be balanced individually to achieve your goals. Variety and specificity work together recursively to benefit each other. With too much specificity, training becomes stale and potentially regressive, while haphazardly selected exercises, volumes, and loads produce equally poor results.

Along with specific movements, consider intensity, volume, density, effort, and lift quality as variables for progression. Tune these to your goals.

Use variety to achieve a broad range of physicality throughout your training career. General Gainz offers multiple forms of progression that help you consistently build momentum—

something real, unlike motivation, a feeling that is ethereal and uncertain. Build momentum by using variation and specificity to propel you forward.

All lifters have bad days. Understand that an increasing frequency of poor workouts signals when it may be time to make some adjustments. Review and evaluate previous workouts to identify potential issues and solutions, including recovery efforts and habits, elements within a single workout, or the progression model itself.

For this reason, diligently track what you do in the gym: weights, reps, sets, effort, rest, and the quality of your movements. This knowledge informs actions:

- Find
- Hold
- Push,
- and Extend

Those <u>Four Actions</u> will guide your progress through the GG framework.

Your data will tell you what lifts to introduce or eliminate. What qualities to focus on (pause, tempo, holds, etc.). What targets to aim for (rep maxes, effort, volume). Knowing these variables, along with others discussed later, yields the best results: a lifetime of sustainable, successful weight training.

"But is General Gainz for hypertrophy or strength?"

Yes.

In the early days of General Gainz, some felt it was less attuned to the needs of a lifter aiming to build size rather than strength. First, gaining strength while eating a surplus of calories will always result in building more muscle. Second, GG inherently includes additional direct training for specific muscle groups: the third tier. Such inclusions will elicit a greater response from those muscles, something you will learn once you are working within this framework.

The sliding scale of variety and specificity does not refer exclusively to generalized movements (e.g., GPP) and specific movements (e.g., the three powerlifts). A program designed to maximize hypertrophy in a particular muscle group can be just as specific as a pure low-rep strength program. It's merely the approach that differs and dictates the result. The General Gainz framework can be adapted to both.

Therefore, if you want to prioritize gaining size over improving your heavy rep maxes, tailor your GG approach to the second and third tiers, limiting or excluding the first tier. On the other end of the spectrum, you could limit T2 and T3 volume, emphasizing heavy rep maxes and their follow-up singles that make up the first tier of GG for a more powerlifting-inspired approach. Of course, a blended approach can also be used: periods that emphasize hypertrophy followed by periods that emphasize strength—periodized training—something GG makes easy to implement.

While training volume is a primary driver of size gains, it is not the be-all and end-all. Effort matters too. As does load. As does time under tension. As does the range of motion. As does rest. The list goes on… Although lifting weights is simple, the biological mechanisms underlying adaptation are complex. Know this: heavy weights do not have to be excluded entirely to achieve hypertrophy. Likewise, it does not require maxing singles or extreme movement specificity to develop maximal strength. Viewing training as a binary relationship unnecessarily limits lifelong growth.

Maximal strength is a skill. It relies on efficient motor unit recruitment and the development of specific movements. These are the emphasis of the first tier. Doing heavier rep maxes and singles with explosive reps will get you stronger, something that is a welcome change of pace after a long period of higher rep, lighter load, grueling bodybuilding-style workouts. But such bodybuilding-inspired workouts lay the foundation for greater strength potential—a simplified way to describe how GG makes it easy to plan, understand, and execute transitions between training phases. These training styles, derived from individual goals, benefit each other.

Developing size and strength is a symbiotic relationship that takes time. Most people, including competitive lifters, bodybuilders, and hobbyists, should implement a periodized training plan to some degree. Such plans benefit overall development by allocating time to areas of need, whether performance or aesthetics, resulting in more well-rounded lifters. For the hobbyist lifter, periodized training plans keep training fresh and interesting: considerable drivers of effort and consistency.

These, and many other reasons I hope to make clear with this book, are why you should consider training using General Gainz for your training.

The Benefit of Volume Drop Sets: CAT

Whereas the commonly used terms "drop sets" or "back-off sets" refer to reducing the weight for subsequent submaximal work after a heavy top set, General Gainz differs by keeping the weight the same while reducing the number of reps per set for additional sets performed with that exercise. In GG, these sets are referred to as "Volume Drop Sets" (VDS).

Example: Following a 6 Rep Max (6RM) with sets of 3 reps (i.e., "Half-Sets") at the same weight.

Put even more simply: You warm up to a 6RM. Rest, then do triples with that weight.

Why this is different: In a 5x5, for example, the load is constrained by the total volume goal of 25 reps. Therefore, the first set will move the fastest, while the last set will move much more slowly than the first.

Here is what makes GG special compared to popular training methods: a 6RM followed by triples means that most of your training volume at that weight is performed explosively, with the total volume comparable to that of a 5x5. That is a critical skill for becoming strong. By using singles and half-sets, you maintain a faster average rep speed for more of your training volume across the first and second tiers. Being powerful with a weight builds size and strength while developing confidence, an intrinsic quality of GG, making it a considerably better approach for nearly everyone.

Your 5RM personal record might crush you. The last rep of the RM will be slow. The next rep? Impossible. A genuine hard effort. However, following that RM with singles opens what I call an "effort gap" (detailed later). In that gap, more volume is completed, developing capacity with that weight. Soon, that weight will be your 6RM. And eventually, your 10RM and more.

Always work to improve a specific skill in the gym. For strength, that skill is force production. So, unless otherwise specified (e.g., tempo or pauses), always perform your Volume Drop Sets as explosively as possible through the concentric range of motion. For aesthetics, that skill might be control. Therefore, be mindful of positioning and rep pacing (colloquially known as the "mind-muscle connection") while maintaining tension in the target muscles.

The emphasis placed on force production is known as "Compensatory Acceleration Training" (CAT) and was popularized long ago by Dr. Fred Hatfield, AKA "Dr. Squat." Although it is an advanced technique, even novice lifters can benefit significantly from it. The goal is to maximize force production without relying solely on load. Be forceful with every rep. Put heavy-weight strength into light weights, moving them explosively, thereby becoming explosive: a characteristic of being strong.

Acceleration increases force production. For that reason, singles and half-sets performed after an RM (moved as explosively as possible) are great for improving force production and thus power and strength. But the same is true for those seeking greater hypertrophy: faster, higher-quality reps mean more effort and more reps, both of which have been shown to build muscle.

Because VDS makes compensatory acceleration easier to practice with GG, know that adding weight to the bar is not the only means of getting stronger. Not only is making your 1RM your 3RM getting stronger, so too is moving a weight faster than before.

Moving fast is a skill worthy of developing. It is a sure way to move more weight and do more reps. This is the essence of training for size and strength.

In summary, Compensatory Acceleration Training (CAT) is a training approach in which the lifter intentionally accelerates the barbell throughout the concentric range of motion, particularly as mechanical advantage increases as the joints near full extension. The goal is to maximize force production by applying more effort even when the weight feels lighter at certain points in the movement.

Key Principles of CAT:

1. **Force Development:** CAT emphasizes producing maximal force with submaximal weights, improving neuromuscular efficiency.

2. **Speed Training:** By accelerating the barbell, lifters develop faster and more powerful contractions, which are essential for explosive movements.

3. **Specificity:** CAT mimics the speed and force requirements of competitive lifts.

4. **Progressive Overload:** CAT allows lifters to practice generating maximal effort without requiring maximal loads, reducing injury risk.

Four Actions: Find, Hold, Push, Extend

Progress in **General Gainz** follows four key actions:

1. **Find**: Increase the weight of the RM or the VDS.

2. **Hold**: Same weight, or reps and sets, and/or rest. (Keeping one or more factors consistent from one week to the next while improving a factor via find, push, or extend.

3. **Push**: More reps per set (RM or VDS) at the same weight, and/or shorter rest periods.

4. **Extend**: More VDS at the same weight with the same reps, or more rest with the same reps.

These actions simplify decision-making during each workout, guiding auto-regulated progression through intensification (weight increases), accumulation (volume increases), density (decreased rest), and quality (better form and consistency across reps and sets).

Examples of these actions during workouts and from week to week are covered later in the discussion of progression models.

Find (Adding Weight – Intensification)

Attempt an RM at a heavier weight—like adding 10 lbs. to your previous 5RM.

- No calculators! Use performance data to guide RM attempts.

- Finding new weights should be earned, not assumed from percentages.

- Over time, repping a weight becomes easier, leading to new Rep Maxes.

- Can be done with the VDS first, if the RM effort is too high to find a heavier weight for the targeted RM. (Example: RM at 315 lbs. with VDS at 325 lbs., next week, RM attempt should be at 325 lbs.)

Hold (Maintaining Performance)

Maintain weight, reps, or sets to increase one while holding the other constant.

- Add weight while maintaining volume (e.g., holding a 5RM at +5 lbs. weekly increase).

- Accumulate volume (e.g., holding 225 lbs. at 5RM while pushing or extending VDS).

- Increase density (e.g., reduce rest while using the same weight and reps as before).

- Ensure control and execution improve before progressing further (qualitative progression).

Push (Adding Volume – Accumulation, or Decreasing Rest)

Increase reps per set or total workout volume.

- Push your RM (e.g., last week's 5RM → this week's 6RM).

- Push Volume Drop Sets (e.g., singles → doubles → triples; turning fives into sixes, going from half-sets to three-quarters in your VDS work).

- Push rest periods shorter, increasing training density.

Avoid pushing weight, volume, and density simultaneously—it's unsustainable.

Extend (Adding Sets or Rest)

Increase Volume Drop Sets beyond the standard limits:

- T1: Up to +3 extra singles beyond the RM value (3RM+6 singles after, maximum).

- T2: Up to six VDS (vs. four standard "half-sets"—fives after a 10RM, for example).

- Only extend if rep quality remains high.

If form deteriorates, consider extending rest instead of sets. Extending rest is also an option if more volume or weight has been added, which may require more recovery time between sets.

Putting It All Together

A simple progression over three weeks:

Week 1: Find a 5RM at 225 lbs. (moderate effort). Follow with sets of 2 reps. Aiming for 4 to 6 sets after the RM.

- **Logged as:** 5RM@225(M) + 2x4

Week 2: Extend VDS to 6.

- **Logged as:** 5RM@225(E) + 2x6

- Note that the effort reduced from moderate to easy because the same weight was used as the week before (the "Hold" action).

Week 3: Push the 5RM to a 6RM.

- **Logged as:** 6RM@225(M) + 3x4

In week four, options include finding an RM at a heavier weight, pushing the same weight for a higher RM, and/or pushing VDS triples to sets of four reps (resulting in VDS being a three-quarter value), extending VDS (limit of 6 sets after the RM), and/or shortening rest.

For example:

Week 4: Find a 5RM at 235 lbs. (moderate effort). Follow with sets of 2 reps. Aiming for 4 to 6 sets after the RM.

- **Logged as:** 5RM@235(M) + 2x4

By cycling **Find, Hold, Push, Extend**, you balance intensity and volume, ensuring steady, sustainable progress.

General Gainz - Terms & Concepts

This list of terms describes specific aspects of General Gainz and how to use it. Each section builds the foundation for the next. Example workouts and programs will be easier to comprehend and adapt if these terms and concepts are well understood.

Training Variables

Progress requires tracking multiple variables. But don't hesitate to deemphasize some, to more effectively emphasize others temporarily. Use variables to fine-tune your training in real time and over a defined period.

If you are performing below expectations, then one or more of these variables may need to be adjusted, including recovery. When these variables are dialed in, consistency improves, resulting in better long-term progress (compared to repeatedly adding weight, for example).

Below are several variables that GG makes easy to consider for both planning and autoregulation. Track these to forecast progress and adjust on the fly when needed.

Intensity: How heavy the work is relative to your one rep max (1RM). The closer the weight is to your one-rep max, the more intense is each rep.

Volume: Is how many reps have been completed with an exercise (and within a workout overall). May also refer to the number of sets for a single exercise or for the entire workout, including all exercises across all tiers.

Effort: The difficulty of a set based on proximity to failure ("reps in reserve"). Was the set easy, moderate, or hard? A hard workout doesn't have to be heavy, nor does an easy workout have to be light or low volume. Effort is independent of both. Effort ratings are discussed in their own section.

Density: How much work is done in a given time, or how long it takes to complete a given workout. Shorter rest intervals between sets result in denser workouts. A dense workout is not necessarily a very intense (heavy) workout. Likewise, a heavy workout made denser over time by reducing rest periods means that the weight is getting less intense: it feels lighter as it moves further from your 1RM (you are getting stronger by getting faster). Improving density is a key factor in enhancing conditioning, therefore work capacity and recovery.

Quality: Posture, speed control, and consistency across sets and workouts. For example, if a lift is "feeling more natural," then you have made qualitative progress. If your reps look similar when your movement pattern was inconsistent before, you've improved quality.

Variation: Variety in movements, intensity, volume, effort, density, and qualities. Along with those, variation is itself a variable. The more variation, the more metrics to track, and the harder it is to discern overall progress. However, variation is often a great means to introduce a novel stimulus, something new to progress, a motivating factor that further drives progress. If training is feeling stale and you have been doing the same lifts for a long time, try increasing exercise variety.

Limiter: A modification to a given lift that reduces the weight and/or effort that can be used, to shift emphasis towards technical execution or a specific muscle (e.g., tempo or pause reps). Another option for exercise variation.

Specificity: Narrowing down the movements, weights, and volumes to more effectively work towards one's goals, turning a template into one's own program. A powerlifter will select competition movements, while a bodybuilder will select movements that favor muscles that build the desired overall body shape.

Further out from a competition, these lifters should incorporate more variety into their training, including lighter loads (for example, "deloads" as commonly found in popular powerlifting programs). This is especially true for novice and intermediate lifters, who should spend more time developing a robust level of physicality through a variety of exercises, loads, and volume.

During the Silver and Golden eras of bodybuilding, lifters trained with a general approach until they neared a show. At that time, "shaping" exercises were added in, further refining the specificity of their training. These changes in variety reflect a simplified periodization approach seen in powerlifting and weightlifting.

Higher specificity enables technical improvements that increase efficiency and, in turn, benefit maximal strength. Likewise, for a bodybuilder who wants to focus on their biceps, training should be structured so that specific movements target the biceps. In this way, specificity can shift from one movement or muscle to another, itself a variable component that progresses independently of others.

Rep Maxes and the First (T1), Second (T2), and Third (T3) Tiers.

A Rep Max (RM) is a measure of how many reps you can perform with a given weight. For example, if you can bench 225 pounds for only one rep, that is your 1RM. Likewise, if you can squat 405 pounds for ten reps, that is your 10RM.

How many reps you can do with a weight determines where it falls within GG's tier scale. That informs how progress can then be made with that exercise and weight. The 1st tier is the heaviest, and thus fewer reps can be completed with such loads. The 2nd tier has moderate weights, allowing more reps. The 3rd tier has the lightest weights, where the most reps are completed in a workout.

These are tiers of a pyramid. The 1st tier, the apex. The 2nd tier, the middle. The 3rd tier, the base. Tiers are based on a spectrum of rep maxes, each with its respective intensity and volume.

When using General Gainz, you will determine your RM ability with a given weight. Once defined, you have several progression options: you can add reps to it ("Pushing" a weight from a lower RM to a higher one), or you can increase that RM by adding weight to it ("Find"). Every T1 and T2 movement should have its own RM. As you train more, you will explore more movements and develop those rep maxes, expanding your exercise repertoire and, in turn, your size and strength.

Though rough approximations can be used by taking a percentage of one applied to the other, it is best to <u>know</u> how many reps you can do with a weight when doing an exercise. Do not use your back squat rep maxes for your front squat; avoid similar overlaps with other lifts. Not sure what your RM is with a movement? Train the lift. Find out. Record your RM sets and the dates. This informs progression, whether adding weight or reps, increasing density, or improving quality.

Rep max sets have an associated effort rating. These are discussed in a later section of this guide.

Bear in mind that hitting a Rep Max does not necessarily imply that a set is performed with maximal effort. Reasonable limits should be in place most of the time. For example, an easier RM with more reps "left in the tank" will allow for more reps to be completed at higher quality via VDS, resulting in improved size and strength. Often, volume is the primary target rather than maximum effort.

Determine your RM less by proximity to muscle failure (and your ability to grind a lift to lockout), and more by a technical standard (your ability to quickly accelerate the bar and produce maximum force). This ensures faster, more powerful reps, while keeping fatigue in check.

Two other common limiters are pauses or slower tempo reps. Keep such limiters and qualities in mind when executing the RM sets. These will result in decreased RMs relative to the weight lifted.

Do not assume that Rep Max always means maximum effort. Remember, effort is a variable itself. Know that your technical limit is a better long-term training standard than lifting to your limit strength.

Technical Limit: The maximum amount of weight lifted with good form.

Limit Strength: The maximum amount of weight lifted, allowing reduced rep quality.

The difference between your limit strength and your technical limit is your injury potential. When you are less skilled in a lift but have a high degree of general strength, that potential is greater. For example, if a person can perform bent-over rows and deadlifts with heavy weight but hasn't practiced the power clean, their injury risk will be higher. The same is true for those who are more skilled at back squats than front squats, and for other lifts with similar overlap.

I mention these because, in such cases, a strong lifter may try a new lift, and while it may move easily, the rep quality is low. Consider this an opportunity to develop skill, and thus quality, rather than aim for intensity or volume progression.

Tier 1 (T1): Heavy Weight Rep Maxes (RM)

Movements:

- Compound lifts: squat, bench, deadlift, press, front squat, snatch, clean, jerk, etc.

Rep Max Range:

- 1RM through 6RM

Volume Drop Sets:

- Singles only (sets of one rep) at the same weight as the RM.

- Performed after the RM. (Exceptions are later detailed.)

Number of Volume Drop Sets to Perform After the RM:

- Goal: Match the RM.

  - Example: 3 singles after a 3RM.

- Extension Limit: +3 additional singles maximum beyond the RM.

  - Example: Up to 6 singles after a 3RM.

- A hard effort RM inherently limits the volume potential for VDS after. Consider extending your singles (T1's Volume Drop Sets) only if the RM effort was easy or moderate.

Volume Ranges for T1 Singles:

This section outlines the volume ranges and suggests courses of action based on performance with that weight. Below are the T1 RMs and recommended singles to complete after the RM, all at the same weight:

- 1RM: Additional singles only if the 1RM was easy. Additional singles are not performed after a moderate or hard effort 1RM. An easy 1RM followed by 1 or 2 more singles is likely a moderate or hard 2 or 3RM.

- 2RM: An additional 1 or 2 more singles can be performed only if the 2RM was easy or moderate. A hard effort 2RM is unlikely to allow for VDS singles.

- 3RM:

    o 1 single = subpar

    o 2 singles = good

    o 3 singles = goal (Even if the 3RM was rated a hard effort, due to the Effort Gap).

    o 4+ singles = attempt RM push in future workouts

        ▪ Singles totaling more than the RM value are considered extended VDS, which in most cases means the RM was rated moderate or easy effort.

- 4RM:

    o 1-2 singles = subpar

- o   3 singles = good
  - o   4 singles = goal
  - o   5+ singles = push RM in the next workout

- 5RM:

  - o   1-3 singles = subpar
  - o   4 singles = good
  - o   5 singles = goal
  - o   6+ singles = push RM in the next workout

- 6RM:

  - o   1-4 singles = subpar
  - o   5 singles = good
  - o   6 singles = goal
  - o   7+ singles = push RM in the next workout

Developing Capacity with a Weight:

- **Subpar performance** means you need to build capacity at this weight by completing more VDS singles in the next workout, within rest limits, before pushing the weight to a higher RM, or finding that RM at a heavier weight.

- To transition a weight from the **T1 to T2** rep range, use it for multiple workouts, increasing VDS singles until you reach the +3 cap beyond the RM. This increases the likelihood of progressing a weight from a 3RM to a 5RM and, eventually, to a 10RM via the push action.

- **Volume cap** (no more than 3 singles beyond RM) prevents excessive work, wasted effort, and unnecessary fatigue.

- When VDS singles feel easy, and volume is fully extended, you can:

  o Increase weight in the next session while maintaining the same RM (**intensification**). E.g., 3RM at 225 lbs. this week to 3 RM at 235 lbs. next week.

  o Push the RM higher with the same weight (e.g., turning a 5RM@225 into a 6RM@225 (**accumulation**).

- While weight increases within a workout are covered in the **Effort Gap** section, remember that when a weight moves easily, you can choose to push it to a higher RM, or push VDS singles to half-sets or half-sets to three-quarters, or progress in another way (density and/or quality) instead of defaulting to adding more weight.

T1 Rest Periods: 3-5 minutes after the RM set, aiming for 2-3 minutes between singles. As capacity improves, 1-2 minutes may be suitable.

Also consider that moderate- and easy-effort RM sets will have a wider effort gap, making the VDS easier and allowing for shorter rest times as a means of densification progression; a great way to develop capacity with T1 weights.

Tier 2 (T2): Middle Weight Rep Maxes (RM)

Movements:

- Compound movements (See T1 examples) and some isolation exercises (e.g., curls).

Rep Max Range:

- 4RM through 10RM.

Volume Drop Sets:

- **"Half" and "Three-Quarter Sets."**
    - **Half-sets:** Each set is ½ of the RM value.
    - **Three-quarter sets:** Each set is ¾ of the RM value.

- Start with half-sets, progressing to three-quarter sets over time via the "push" action.

- This approach develops work capacity and enables a successful RM push later.

- Volume Drop Sets do not have to be the same value across all sets:
    - Example: Start with half-sets and, if feeling good, push the last set to three-quarters.
    - If operating in the bridge weight range, adjust reps from triples to doubles or even singles if needed.

- Increasing reps per VDS is accumulation, meaning you're adding training volume to a weight, pushing it across the bridge from the heavier end to the lighter end. For example, if you push moderate 5RM weight to a hard 6RM, you might be able to start with doubles but perhaps feel strong enough in the last few sets to go for triples.

- Decreasing reps per VDS is intensification, meaning you're going the opposite way by adding weight, moving from the lighter end to the heavier end of the bridge, for example, if you found a new hard effort 5RM and started its VDS as doubles but ended up finishing the sets at singles.

Effort-Based Adjustments:

- **Hard effort RM:** Consider reducing reps in Volume Drop Sets to reduce fatigue.

  - Example: After a **hard 5RM**, perform **one rep per sets** (singles) instead of half-sets. After the first one or two singles, you might feel confident enough (and recovered enough from the RM) to make the remaining VDS into doubles.

- This helps manage fatigue, allowing for more total Volume Drop Sets and greater capacity development. So, perhaps your goal was 4 three-quarter sets after a 10RM; instead, you completed only two sets of seven reps, followed by a set of six, and a final set of five reps.

- **Easy effort RM:** Consider increasing reps in the VDS.

  - Perform three-quarter sets instead of half-sets for all, or a portion of the VDS.

  - Example: After an **easy 5RM**, perform **three reps per set** instead of doubles or singles (singles would indicate that the 5RM was harder than rated and/or your work capacity at that weight is more aligned with the T1).

- This develops skill and builds capacity with that weight.

Number of Volume Drop Sets to Perform After the RM:

- **Goal:** Double the volume of the Rep Max. Extend up to 6 VDS after your RM to build more capacity, making an RM push more likely (e.g., when you attempt to make your 5RM a 6+RM).

- **Typically:** Four half-sets (start here, extend up to six when needed).

  - If performing three-quarter sets, complete fewer total sets. Only extend the three-quarter value VDS to five or six sets if the RM is stubborn and proving very difficult to push to a higher RM value.

- **Examples:**

  - **Half-set approach:** 10RM + **5 reps x 4 sets** (20 VDS reps after a 10RM).

  - **Three-quarter set approach:** 10RM + **7 reps x 3 sets** (21 VDS reps after a 10RM).

    - The three-quarter approach has a narrower Effort Gap, so that rep quality will be more challenging, but when training to push high RM sets even higher, this method of building capacity will be needed.

    - Three-quarter VDS can be extended to six sets total but start with three sets.

- **Three-quarter sets narrow the effort gap,** making them more challenging and fatiguing.

- **For newly found T2 weights:**

  - Start with half-sets.

  - Push VDS to three-quarter sets in later workouts, if in an accumulation cycle. Reduce from half-sets to singles as the RM decreases during an intensification cycle.

  - Accumulation allows you to push the RM further into the T2 rep range and beyond, eventually into the T3 range if desired. In contrast, intensification requires reducing half-sets to singles as the RM decreases while increasing the weight from workout to workout.

Extension Limit:

- **+2 additional half or three-quarter sets** beyond the standard four, meaning, five to six T2 VDS is the limit.

Volume Ranges for T2 follow-up half- and three-quarter Volume Drop Sets:

RM	Reps per Set	Sets	Extended Set Limit
4	2-3	3-4	6
5	2-3	3-4	6
6	2-4	3-4	6
7	3-5	3-4	6
8	4-6	3-4	6
9	4-7	3-4	6
10	5-8	3-4	6
11+	6-9	3-4	6

Increasing Capacity and Workload

Weights around a 10RM are entering the T3 range—lighter loads that allow for higher reps. Because of this, half-sets create a wider effort gap, allowing for multiple progression options, such as:

- Three-quarter value VDS.

- Increasing training density by reducing rest

- Performing supersets

- Incorporating tempo or paused reps

Assessing Volume Drop Sets:

- **1–2 sets after the RM → Subpar**: The RM was likely too difficult, indicating a lack of capacity or technical proficiency. Reduce the weight for that RM in your next session to allow for more Volume Drop Sets.

- **3 sets after the RM → Good**: Solid performance, showing progress.

- **4 sets after the RM → Goal**: Ideal workload for capacity building.

- **5–6 sets after the RM → Extended Range**: If you can complete this, your RM was likely rated as "easy" or "moderate," especially if using three-quarter sets instead of half-sets.

Building Work Capacity:

- If you've reached 5–6 Volume Drop Sets, you're likely ready to push that weight from a lower-rep RM to a higher-rep RM, or add weight while holding that target RM.

- If rest times were generous, start reducing them to increase training density and further improve work capacity.

By systematically progressing Volume Drop Sets and managing rest, you'll be able to move weights from the heavier end of T2 into the lighter ranges of T3, reinforcing long-term strength and endurance gains through accumulation (adding volume via push and extend actions) or intensification (adding weight via the find action) as you progress a movement from the T2 into the T1.

When training a lift in the T2 range, perhaps starting at 6RM and adding weight weekly until that movement reaches 1RM, increase rest between sets as the load increases, necessitating your VDS decrease from triples to doubles to singles.

T2 Rest Periods: 2 to 3 minutes after the RM set, aiming for 1 to 2 minutes between half- and three-quarter-sets.

T1 & T2 Bridge Weights (Moving a weight between the T1 & T2)

The 4RM, 5RM, and 6RM are Bridge Weights that overlap between T1 and T2. At these loads, capacity expands beyond singles, allowing Volume Drop Sets to be a mix of singles (T1) and half-sets (T2).

- **Effort determines VDS approach:**

    o   Hard RM effort? Stick to singles for better quality and bar speed.

    o   Easy or moderate RM effort? Half-sets may be a better option.

    o   A mix of both is also possible—start with half-sets and switch to singles if needed.

Progressing a Bridge Weight

- Begin with **singles** after a 4RM.

- While holding the same 4RM target and weight, progress to doubles, pushing the singles into half-sets (accumulation) the next week.

- Once all VDS volumes consist of half-sets, the weight has moved from **T1 → T2**.

    o   Pushing a weight from the heavy side of the bridge to the lighter side.

- Over time, the RM increases, e.g., a **4RM → 5RM → 6RM**, pushing the weight deeper into T2. Eventually, it will become a T3 weight. This happens via the Four Actions.

Example Accumulation Progression:

1. **Week 1:** 5RM (Hard effort) + 1 rep x 5 sets (singles).

2. **Week 2:** Using the same weight and performing another 5RM, extend singles to 8 sets.

3. **Week 3:** 5RM → 6RM + a mix of singles and doubles as the VDS.

4. **Week 4:** Hold the 6RM. All VDS are pushed to double. This weight is now a T2.

5. **Week 5+:** 6RM → 8RM, continuing to push the VDS and the RM in an alternating manner.

Example Accumulation Progression:

1. **Week 1:** 5RM (Easy effort) + 3 reps x 4 sets.

2. **Week 2:** Add weight. The RM becomes a moderate effort. Triples become doubles.

3. **Week 3:** Add weight. The RM is now a hard effort. Doubles become singles.

4. **Week 4:** Add weight. The 5RM reduces to a moderate 4RM, allowing for up to 7 singles.

Key Rule: Let rep quality guide volume. If singles feel easy, switch to doubles/triples as that movement's last VDS in that workout, or as the VDS in the next workout.

Tier 3 (T3): Light Weight Rep Maxes (RM) and Rep Ranges

T3 exercises include **accessory lifts** (isolation or compound) that serve different goals:

1. **Strength Support**: Strengthen muscles needed for T1/T2 lifts (e.g., leg extensions for squats, pec fly for bench, row for deadlift).

2. **Technique Development**: Refine movement patterns (e.g., single-leg RDLs for deadlift).

3. **Muscle Growth**: Focus on hypertrophy (e.g., biceps curls and delt raises for aesthetics).

4. **Prehab/Rehab**: Support joint health and injury prevention (e.g., grip and rotator cuff work post injury).

There is no "optimal" selection. Choose movements based on your goals and experiment with them.

For example, if you are in an accumulation phase with more bodybuilding-inspired goals, do more T3s that target the desired muscle groups. Or, if you're in an intensification phase with more powerlifting-inspired goals, include T3s that support the squat, bench, and deadlift, such as leg press, close-grip bench, and hyperextensions.

Rep & Volume Guidelines

- **Standard T3 rep ranges:**

  o **15–20 reps** per set (3–4 sets)

  o **12–15 reps** per set (3–4 sets)

- o **10–12 reps** per set (3–4 sets)

- o **8–10 reps** per set (3–4 sets)

- **Heavier T3 ranges** (end of blocks, "Crossing the bridge" training a lift to become a potential T2 movement):

  - o **6–8 reps** per set (2–3 sets)

  - o **5–7 reps** per set (2–3 sets)

The T3 can follow either an intensification or an accumulation progression. However, because of the higher rep nature of the T3, it will typically follow an intensification progression, adding weight each week while gradually working towards lower rep ranges; this can be the case even when T1 and T2 are themselves in an accumulation phase

The primary reason is to avoid adding volume across all lifts and tiers simultaneously. However, after an intensification phase (such as a peaking cycle), accumulating volume in the T3 first is a great way to rebuild any lost work capacity from the volume decline during such a cycle. This need is based on the effort target and your recovery needs.

Progression & Execution

- **All sets are for Max Rep Sets (MRS):** First set aims for the high end of the rep range, with reps naturally decreasing due to fatigue (e.g., **15/13/12** for a **12–15 rep range**).

- **Each set is performed to a target effort:** Easy, Moderate, or Hard.

    o   Increasing or lowering the weight between sets to stay within the targeted range is allowed. However, it may not be needed. Do not adjust the weight between sets merely to stay at the top end of the range; allow a slight decrease in reps while staying within the range and maintaining effort.

- **Total volume per movement:** 30–60 reps across 3–4 sets, allowing for a margin of a handful of reps. If +/- 5 reps from this total rep range, the weight was too light or too heavy for the movement and targeted rep range. Account for this in future workouts.

- **T3 can transition into T2:**

    o   If progressing a T3 lift towards T2, gradually increase weight and lower reps over time, finding that lift in the 5-8 reps per set range. At this point, this lift can be trained within the T2, following those load and rep progression guidelines.

    o   Example: A movement that starts as **12/11/10/10 (43 reps total)** can become heavier, going to **10/9/8/8 (35 reps total)** by adding weight, eventually becoming a T2 RM followed by half-sets (e.g., 7RM(M)+4 reps x4-6 sets). This is the process of intensification.

Key Considerations

- **Adjust volume based on work capacity**: Hard-effort sets can be fatiguing. If your program calls for a week of hard-effort T3s, you may end up doing only 1 to 2 sets.

- **Not every set needs to be maximal effort**: Leave some reps in reserve when necessary. This may depend on where you're at in a training cycle and/or your recovery needs; easier sets are easier to recover from. Apply effort ratings to your T3 and use them as a progression variable.

- **Experiment with progression strategies**: Find what works best for your goals. E.g., rest-pause method or keeping a lift in the heavier range versus lighter because you found it responded better to the lower-volume end of the T3; lat pull-downs, for example.

Alternate T3 Progression Option

Instead of rep ranges, consider **total rep targets** for T3 exercises. Once the target is met, increase the weight. This is volume accumulation in the T3 range.

- Keep the weight constant and perform sets until you've accumulated the **minimum rep target** (e.g., **60 reps in 3–4 sets**).

- Common targets: **60, 45, or 30 reps** in **2–4 sets per exercise**.

- o Example: Performing sets of 12/10/9/8 for a total of 39 reps, then, using the same weight the next week, add reps, perhaps doing 14/12/11/9 (46 reps).

- Fewer sets (e.g., 2) occur when sets are **hard effort**, reaching **15–20 reps** with a lighter weight.

T3 Rest Periods: 30 to 90 seconds between MRS.

T2 & T3 Bridge Weights (Transitioning Between T2 & T3)

The **9RM, 10RM, and 11RM** act as **Bridge Weights** between **T2 and T3**.

- Accumulation: Making a T2 half-set a three-quarter VDS, then as the weight feels lighter because of building capacity, that three-quarter VDS can become an MRS. This way, your RM is followed by sets of max reps, per the T3 guidance above.

- Intensification: Making the first set of a T3 MRS an RM, and doing three-quarter value VDS afterwards, eventually, by adding weight, those become half-sets as that lift transitions from T3 to T2 and perhaps a T1 if appropriate.

  - o For example, if training a new compound lift, like Zerchers, which can take a while to get used to. Zerchers are great to start in the T3 but can be trained well in the T1 after skill (and pain tolerance) has been developed.

Confirming the T3 Transition:

Accumulation: If you can complete six three-quarter VDS, repeat the workout, performing each set as an MRS. This confirms that the weight has shifted from T2 to T3 territory.

Intensification: If, after the first MRS of around 10 to 12 reps, the next set is three or four reps less. In this case, the lift would be better trained following the T2 guidance, performing a three-quarter or half-set value VDS.

Strategies to Close the Effort Gap in the T2 and T3:

- Push half-sets → three-quarter sets.

- Reduce rest time.

- Use super sets, tempo work, or paused reps for added stimulus.

- Once the effort gap becomes too wide (such as an easy 12RM followed by 6 sets of 8 reps), train the weight as a T3, focusing on higher reps per set using MRS instead of VDS.

By following these steps, you systematically push weights from **T1 → T3** and vice versa, ensuring continuous progression.

Bodyweight Exercise Considerations

Bodyweight exercises can be assigned to any tier (T1, T2, or T3) depending on strength level and training goals. Stronger lifters have more options, but all athletes can effectively program bodyweight movements.

T3 Placement (Most Common)

- Exercises like pull-ups, push-ups, dips, sit-ups, and leg lifts are often trained in T3.

- They can be done with either of the T3 approaches described above.

T1 & T2 Placement (For Lower Reps)

- If you struggle to perform 10 reps in one set, treat the exercise as T1 or T2 and follow an accumulation progression to build reps using only bodyweight.

- Example progression if you can only do 4 pull-ups:

    o **T1:** Perform an RM followed by singles afterwards.

    o **T2:** Use half-sets after your RM, progress these to three-quarter VDS.

    o **T3:** Once three-quarter VDS are consistent and easy, transition to MRS.

Example: Training Pull-ups

- Lifter with a 10-rep max of pull-ups, for example:

- o **T2 Approach:** Do a 10RM + six sets of five reps for 40 total reps (higher volume without near-max fatigue due to the effort gap), practicing qualitative aspects like pauses, holds, or slow eccentrics. Consider adding a small amount of weight to the half-sets, as this will develop your RM ability with bodyweight, pushing it further into the T3, where you can do MRS instead of VDS.

  - o **T3 Approach:** Perform 4 MRS at an easy effort, e.g., 10/9/8/7 (34 reps total, low-end T3 volume). Try adding reps as able to each of these sets weekly, building up to 40 or more reps over time.

Tempo Manipulation for Progression

- Slow eccentrics (3–4 sec) help maintain effort across tiers and improve execution.

  - o Example: If 15–20 leg lifts are too easy at a normal rep tempo, slow the eccentric or add holds at the top/bottom of the range.

By adjusting tier placement, rep schemes, and tempo, bodyweight exercises can be effectively integrated into the General Gainz framework.

Volume Table

General Gainz

Rep Max	RM	Follow-Up Reps	Follow-Up Sets
First Tier (T1)	1	Singles	**Match RM. Extension limit = +3 beyond RM.** Example: 3 to 6 singles after a 3RM.
	2	Singles	
	3	Singles	
	4	Singles or Half-Sets	**Bridge Weights** — If RM is moderate or easy effort, perform 2s or 3s (half-sets). If RM is hard effort, perform singles. Mix as needed across all follow-up sets.
	5	Singles or Half-Sets	
Second Tier (T2)	6	Singles or Half-Sets	
	7	Half-Sets	**4 sets after the RM. Extension limit = 6.**
	8	Half-Sets	
	9	Half-, Three-Quarter, or Max Rep Sets	**Bridge Weights** — If Half- or Three-Quarter, **4 to 6 sets.** If MRS (T3) then **3 to 4 sets.**
	10		
Third Tier (T3)	11+	Max Rep Sets (MRS)	

Reps per set are flexible. Not all follow-up sets have to be the same value. Adjust based on rep quality.

Example: After a 7RM the first few sets may be 4s and the last few 3s.

Effort Guide **Easy: 2+ Reps in Reserve** **Apply effort rating to RM sets. If RM is**
Moderate: 1 Rep in Reserve **skipped, then effort is applied to the first and**
Hard: 0 Reps in Reserve **last set of singles and/or half-sets.**

Lift within technical limit. Do not push all RM sets to max effort. Effort guides volume, intensity, quality, and density. Each are related. Read General Gainz to learn these relationships.

Rest Guide T1: 3 to 5 min. after RM. 2 to 3 min./follow-up singles.
T2: 2 to 3 min. after RM. 1 to 2 min./follow-up sets.
T3: 30 to 90 seconds between sets.

Less rest requires lower loads and/or easier efforts with higher quality reps.

Increase density (less rest) between follow-up sets to build capacity for finding new (heavier) RM weights and/or pushing RM weights higher (in effect, making those weights lighter).

Use the table above to determine which rep and progression scheme to follow after an RM. Progression works best when you reach the "Goal" volume for Volume Drop Sets. "Good" works, but if you find a lift stalling, try performing more volume.

At various points in their lifetimes, lifts will require different volumes depending on your goals and your ability with those lifts. For example, if the squat is your primary goal, keep VDS in the "Goal" range (four sets), possibly extending to six sets when able, while keeping deadlift in the "Good" range (three sets); consider the same for bench and press.

Be deliberate with your volume. Don't always maximize it for the sake of merely doing more.

Rest Times

Rest periods are a crucial part of the General Gainz structure. Without them, an endless number of Volume Drop Sets could be performed, making density progression—and therefore work capacity development—impossible. Rest itself is a form of progression.

By gradually reducing rest times, you can close the effort gap between Volume Drop Sets, allowing you to turn a 5RM into a 10RM, then a 20RM. This requires patience and consistency as you develop strength-endurance.

Rest Guidelines

Rest times should adjust based on effort. If a 5RM feels easy but you still prefer singles over half-sets, shortening rest periods is a smart move. Reducing rest before increasing volume is a cautious and practical approach.

- **T1 Lifts:** 3–5 minutes after the RM set, with 2–3 minutes between singles.

- **T2 Lifts:** 2–3 minutes after the RM set, with 1–2 minutes between half-sets.

- **T3 Lifts:** 30–90 seconds between MRS.

If a new RM PR leaves you gassed, rest more between follow-up VDS. Over time, gradually reduce rest to implement density progression. If your RM was easy, your rest times can be shorter; this is a good means to improve capacity with that weight.

Barbell Warm-up

This is my warm-up protocol for all main movements (any compound barbell exercise). Adjust the loads based on the weight you plan to work up to for your RM.

If your deadlift target is a 3RM at 600 pounds, you will make larger increases in weight earlier in the warm-up progression as you perform sets working towards 600 pounds. Conversely, if your working weight is lower, let's say you're overhead pressing 135 pounds for a 5RM, then you will make smaller increases between warm-up sets.

As an example, a lifter with estimated 5RMs of 385-pound squat, 245-pound bench, and 425-pound deadlift would work up to those weights in such a manner:

Squat:
95x10, 135x5, 185x5, 225x3, 275x3, 315x1, 365x1, 385x [RM + Volume Drop Sets]

Bench:
45x10, 95x5, 135x5, 165x3, 185x3, 205x1, 225x1, 235x1, 245x [RM + Volume Drop Sets]

Deadlift:
135x10, 225x5, 275x3, 315x3, 365x1, 405x1, 425x [RM + Volume Drop Sets]

Note that the deadlift has fewer warm-up reps, whereas the bench has more. This is fine! Not every lift requires the same reps per set, the same total warm-up sets, or the same increases from set to set. Personally speaking, I warm up quickly and easily when deadlifting. Other lifts may take longer to get into the groove. Your experience may be different; for example, I know many lifters who do 2 or 3 sets at a light weight (such as 225 from the above progression), as it helps them get the movement dialed in while keeping effort and thus fatigue very low.

The closer the warm-up sets are to the working weight, the smaller the weight increases and the fewer the reps per set; thus, the reduction to singles as you approach the weight being lifted for the RM. Adjust the increments as you see fit. The objective is to perform 5 to 8 sets, progressing to the targeted weight and RM.

These sets generally use 25- and 45-pound plates, but for lighter lifts, such as the bench press, overhead press, and row, you will do better with smaller jumps from warm-up set to warm-up set, allowing for a more thorough warm-up and facilitating a successful, productive workout. This is more true for newer lifters and those whose strength is at lower weight thresholds.

Full Example Sessions

The following workouts illustrate how T1, T2, and T3 exercises fit into a single session. These are just examples—your actual training will be part of a larger progression tailored to your goals, needs, and abilities.

General Structure

- **T1:** One primary lift per session (e.g., squat, bench, deadlift, press).

- **T2:** One to two complementary exercises (e.g., front squat, close grip bench, barbell rows, and incline bench press).

- **T3:** Three to six accessory exercises (depending on lifter capacity).

Exceptions & Variations

- **Powerlifters & Strength Athletes:** May include two T1 lifts if training frequency is lower, perhaps training only 3x per week (e.g., squat & bench in the same session). T2 exercises would complement these lifts (e.g., pause squats or Romanian deadlifts, and close-grip or incline bench).

- **Bodybuilding Focus:** Might exclude T1 singles, doing only the RM sets, and focus more on the T2 and T3 to allow for higher training volume, density, and shorter rest periods.

- **Conditioning-Oriented Workouts:** Prioritize density and higher reps and T3 movements with minimal rest. These are often paired with T2 exercises and/or cardio, such as benching with 100 meters of rowing on the erg between bench VDS.

The following examples illustrate different workout structures for various training styles. Use them as inspiration, adapting them to fit your broader progression and individual goals.

General Strength

Example Workout A (Leg & Back Focus)

T1 (Primary Lift)

- **Squat**: 5RM @ [Working Weight] (Effort Rating)

- Followed by **+1 rep** x **5 to 8 sets** (based on effort)

  - Example: 5RM@225(M)+1x5-8

T2 (Supplementary Lift)

- **Romanian Deadlift**: 10RM @ [Working Weight] (Effort Rating)

- Followed by **+5 to 8 reps** x **4 to 6 sets** (based on effort)

  - Example: 10RM@315(E)+5x4-6

T3 (Accessory Lifts – Max Rep Sets)

- **T3a: Barbell Row**: [Target Rep Range] x 3-4 sets (Easy/Moderate/Hard Effort)

  - Example: 10-12 reps @Moderate Effort. Result: 12/11/10/10

- **T3b: Leg Press**: [Target Rep Range] x 3-4 sets (Easy/Moderate/Hard Effort)

  - Example: 10-12 reps @Moderate Effort. Result: 12/12/11/10

- **T3c: Lat Pulldown**: [Target Rep Range] x 3-4 sets (Easy/Moderate/Hard Effort)

    o Example: 12-15 reps @Moderate Effort. Result: 15/14/12/12

Workout Execution & Progression

This workout prioritizes leg and back development through a structured progression model:

- **T1:** Performed at the upper end of the range (5RM), followed by singles if at moderate or hard effort. (If the effort was easy, this has the potential to be a T1/T2 bridge weight by including some doubles with the singles.)

- **T2:** Also begins at the upper range (10RM). Effort rating after the RM set determines VDS—adjusting half-sets to three-quarter sets (thus 5 to 8 reps per set) or extending total volume (by performing five to six sets after the RM).

- **T3:** Executed as Max Rep Sets (MRS) within a target rep range (e.g., 10-12 and 12–15 reps). The load should be adjusted to maintain consistency of effort and movement across sets.

Progression Strategy (Find / Hold / Push / Extend)

When repeating this workout:

- **T1:** Hold a 5RM target while finding a heavier weight. Continue performing VDS as singles.

- **T2:** Push and/or extend VDS while maintaining the same weight from the last session.

- **T3:** Push last week's weight to a higher rep range while holding the same weight (accumulation) or add weight to those exercises and reduce the reps per set as needed (intensification).

This structured approach ensures continuous adaptation while effectively managing fatigue and effort.

Example Workout B (Upper Body Focus)

T1 (Primary Lift)

- **Bench Press**: 3RM @ [Working Weight] (Effort Rating)

- Followed by **+1 rep** x **3 to 6 sets** (based on effort)
    - Example: 3RM@295(H)+1x3-6

T2 (Supplementary Lift)

- **Incline Bench Press**: 7RM @ [Working Weight] (Effort Rating)

- Followed by **+3 to 5 reps** x **4 to 6 sets** (based on effort)
    - Example: 7RM@175(M)+4x4-6

T3 (Accessory Lifts – Max Rep Sets)

- **T3a: Arnold Press** – [Target Rep Range] x 3-4 sets (Easy/Moderate/Hard Effort)

    o   Example: 8-10 reps @Moderate Effort. Result: 10/9/8/8

- **T3b: Lateral Raise** – [Target Rep Range] x 3-4 sets (Easy/Moderate/Hard Effort)

    o   Example: 8-10 reps @Moderate Effort. Result: 10/10/10/9

- **T3c: Triceps Extension** – [Target Rep Range] x 3-4 sets (Easy/Moderate/Hard Effort)

    o   Example: 8-10 reps @Moderate Effort. Result: 10/9/9/8

Progression Strategy

- For both T1 & T2 VDS, the total volume after the RM depends on its effort.

- To accumulate volume, start at the lower end of the volume range and increase reps or sets as capacity allows.

    o   **Push & Extend:** Add volume by extending T1 singles to the +3 limit beyond the RM. For T2, push the rep ranges (half-sets → three-quarter sets) or extend VDS to 5 or 6 total.

- To increase intensity, add weight while trying to hold volume (RM and VDS), allowing effort to increase according to the amount of weight added to the exercise.

Key Considerations

- Easy or moderate RM efforts allow for volume increases within and between workouts.

- Hard RM efforts may limit VDS. E.g., an 8RM at hard effort likely won't allow six sets of six reps (three-quarter sets, fully extended). The better option, if aiming for volume development, would be four reps per set over four to six sets.

- Progression can involve:

  o Holding T1 & T2 RM targets while increasing weight ("Find" action).

  o Adding VDS based on effort and capacity ("Extend" action).

  o Recognizing differences in capacity across lifts (e.g., higher bench press capacity vs. overhead pressing) so you're adding weight to one while adding reps to another.

The goal is to gradually increase weight or volume (intensification or accumulation) across repeated workouts while managing fatigue and effort.

Powerlifting

Example Workout A (Lower Body Focus)

T1a: Squat 3RM @ [Working Weight] (Effort Rating) +1 rep x 3 to 6 sets

T1b: Bench 3RM@ [Working Weight] (Effort Rating) +1 rep x 3 to 6 sets

T2: Deficit Deadlift 6RM@ [Working Weight] (Effort Rating) +2 to 4 reps x 4 to 6 sets

T3a: Split Squat [Target Rep Range] x 3-4 sets (Easy/Moderate/Hard Effort)

T3b: Quadriceps Extension [Target Rep Range] x 3-4 sets (Easy/Moderate/Hard Effort)

T3c: Hamstring Curl [Target Rep Range] x 3-4 sets (Easy/Moderate/Hard Effort)

Powerlifting-Focused Workout Structure

This workout includes two T1 exercises (squat and bench) to prioritize powerlifting performance. Squat and bench could be superset, but let fatigue guide. Super-setting T2 deadlifts with T1b bench presses could work, but T1a squats with T2 deadlifts would fatigue each other, limiting performance. All that said, supersets are generally unnecessary.

While powerlifting doesn't require high-frequency training, some lifters benefit from increased frequency when preparing for a meet. This could be one of multiple weekly sessions featuring squat, bench press, and deadlift variations.

The T2 and T3 exercises focus on lower-body development. The next session might emphasize upper-body work, including both chest and back.

Progression Strategy

- Prioritize adding weight while maintaining volume, reducing RM targets as the weight increases weekly. Keep in mind that the VDS will also decrease gradually, in proportion to the RM achieved.

- Hold volume as long as possible before increasing weight to the point where full volume can't be sustained. This will increase effort between workouts, as you will be finding the same RM at a heavier weight. Once an RM is achieved at a hard effort, add weight the next week, allowing yourself to reduce the target RM, as you near a 1RM attempt.

- Adjust movement selection based on skill, ability, and training schedule. If you are preparing for a meet, it is best to use lifts you are skilled at, as those will allow the most work to be done, whereas less-trained lifts would require lighter loads, thereby limiting the training stimulus necessary to develop maximal strength for powerlifting.

Example Workout B (Upper Body Focus)

T1a: Deadlift 3RM @ [Working Weight] (Effort Rating) +1 rep x 3 to 6 sets

T1b: Long-Pause Bench 5RM@ [Working Weight] (Effort Rating) +1 rep x 3 to 6 sets

T2: Incline Bench Press 6RM@ [Working Weight] (Effort Rating) +2 to 4 reps x 4 to 6 sets

T3a: DB Bench [Target Rep Range] x 3-4 sets (Easy/Moderate/Hard Effort)

T3b: Pec Fly [Target Rep Range] x 3-4 sets (Easy/Moderate/Hard Effort)

T3c: Triceps Push Down [Target Rep Range] x 3-4 sets (Easy/Moderate/Hard Effort)

Powerlifting Workout B – Deadlift Focus

This workout complements Workout A by shifting the T1 focus to deadlifts and including a lighter bench press variation. This setup allows for:

- A heavy deadlift day, with Workout A serving as the lighter deadlift session.

- A second lighter T1 bench press, enabling better pause training and increased volume (extending up to 8 singles after a 5RM, based on effort). Then pushing singles to doubles – crossing the bridge (accumulation wave).

Effort Gap & Training Adaptations

- RM sets may be performed at regular tempo, while VDS are paused to increase difficulty and close the effort gap.

- T3 exercises in this session prioritize the upper body, specifically for bench press performance. Other sessions during the week may focus on squats (legs) or deadlifts (back).

Progression Strategy – Intensification Phase

- Hold volume while adding weight each session.

- If adding weight reduces rep quality, adjust reps per set of VDS accordingly to reprioritize skill development via quality (going from triples to doubles to singles, for example).

- Gradually progress T3 exercises, scaling volume as work capacity allows.

Caution Against Rapid Weight Increases

- Avoid increasing weight too quickly, which forces a rapid volume drop, useful for meet prep but not ideal mid-cycle.

Bodybuilding

Example Workout A (Legs)

T1a: Squat 10RM @ [Working Weight] (Effort Rating) +5 to 8 reps x 4 to 6 sets

T1b: Romanian Deadlift 10RM@ [Working Weight] (Effort Rating) +5 to 8 reps x 4 to 6 sets

T3a: Hack Squat [Target Rep Range] x 3-4 sets (Easy/Moderate/Hard Effort)

T3b: Leg Curls [Target Rep Range] x 3-4 sets (Easy/Moderate/Hard Effort)

T3c: Leg Extensions [Target Rep Range] x 3-4 sets (Easy/Moderate/Hard Effort)

T3d: Calf Raise [Target Rep Range] x 3-4 sets (Easy/Moderate/Hard Effort)

Leg Day in the GG Framework

This balanced leg day includes both anterior and posterior chain exercises, but you can adjust the focus as desired:

- To bias the anterior chain, swap leg curls for walking lunges and calf raises for tibialis raises.

- To bias the posterior chain, swap hack squats for hip thrusts and leg extensions for back-step lunges

- Modify exercises based on individual goals to emphasize specific muscles.

Bodybuilding Approach

- T1 exercises are generally excluded in a bodybuilding-focused GG workout.

- While heavy lifting has benefits, higher volume yields better muscle growth relative to fatigue and risk exposure due to limited T1 training. Don't randomly throw T1 reps into a bodybuilding wave. Spend a wave building up, as this will develop your skill and strength potential at those much heavier intensities.

- Focus effort on T2 and T3 movements for hypertrophy. Keep the RM effort targets higher, at moderate or hard (1 or 0 RiR). Apply an effort-gap-closing quality, such as supersets, when appropriate. T3 effort should be higher compared to a powerlifting-focused plan.

Training Density & Supersets

- Supersets increase density, but do them without sacrificing rep quality. Example pairings:

    o Leg Extension + Leg Curls

- Supersets aren't inherently superior for muscle growth, but can be a fun and efficient option, while reducing your time in the gym.

Example Workout B (Chest & Triceps)

T2a: Military Press 10RM@ [Working Weight] (Effort Rating) +5 to 8 reps x 4 to 6 sets

T2b: Incline Bench 10RM@ [Working Weight] (Effort Rating) +5 to 8 reps x 4 to 6 sets

T3a: DB Bench Press [Target Rep Range] x 3-4 sets (Easy/Moderate/Hard Effort)

T3b: Pec Fly [Target Rep Range] x 3-4 sets (Easy/Moderate/Hard Effort)

T3c: Triceps Kickback [Target Rep Range] x 3-4 sets (Easy/Moderate/Hard Effort)

T3d: Triceps Push Down [Target Rep Range] x 3-4 sets (Easy/Moderate/Hard Effort)

Upper Body Push Day in the GG Framework

This workout targets upper-body pushing muscles as part of a push-pull-legs split within a GG framework-built program. Since there are no back exercises here, a pull-focused workout can be scheduled for the following day or two, then resume with legs.

T3 Volume & Customization

- Four T3 exercises are included for simplicity, but more can be added if time and recovery allow.

- Additional lateral raises or isolation work can be included based on individual goals. Personally, I need to bomb my delts to make them grow. When running a Push, Pull, Legs split on a 6x weekly training schedule, I like my second Push day to be more shoulder-focused; this is when I do lateral raises.

Fatigue Considerations

- GG's Max Rep Set (MRS) approach is more fatiguing than standard 3x10 training. That said, adjust the load between sets to stay within the target rep range at the desired effort level.

- Beginners should start conservatively with intensity and effort before increasing volume.

Progression for Bodybuilding

- Use accumulation-based progression:

    o Hold the same weight and push 10RM toward 15-20RM before adding weight.

    o Increase T3 rep targets (with the same weight) before increasing load.

    o Once volume goals are reached, reset with heavier weight and lower reps, then repeat.

This method biases time under tension, improves work capacity, and reduces injury risk, ensuring consistent muscle growth over time. Add weight and/or reps per previous guidance.

Conditioning:

Example Workout A (Fixed Time, Variable Work)

60 Minutes, As Many Rounds/Reps As Possible

Giant Set / Circuit

Guidance: Super Set the Squat VDS with the T3 MRS.

T2a: Squat 10RM@ [Working Weight] (Effort Rating) +5 to 8 reps x 4 to 6 sets

[Super Set] T3a: Pull-ups @Bodyweight x Max Reps x 3 to 6 Sets (Easy/Moderate/Hard Effort)

[Super Set] T3b: RDL [Target Rep Range] x 3-4 sets (Easy/Moderate/Hard Effort)

[Super Set] T3c: Press [Target Rep Range] x 3-4 sets (Easy/Moderate/Hard Effort)

[Super Set] T3d: Sit-ups [Target Rep Range] x 3-4 sets (Easy/Moderate/Hard Effort)

[Super Set] T3e: Farmers Walk [Target Rep Range] x 3-4 sets (Easy/Moderate/Hard Effort)

Fixed-Time Conditioning Workout (GG Framework)

In this density-driven workout, you aim to complete as much work as possible within a set time. You cycle through exercises, T2 squats, pull-ups, RDLs, etc., repeating that cycle until time runs out. The number of sets (or rounds) is the variable, with a challenging but achievable upper limit.

Workout Structure & Flexibility

- Includes one T2 (in this case the squat) and five T3 exercises for full-body conditioning.

- It can be scaled to focus on fewer muscle groups based on goals, stamina, and ability.

- A giant set format minimizes rest, but if your gym setup doesn't allow circuits, perform each exercise separately with minimal rest (consider a quarter-set density approach).

Effort & Rep Considerations

- Lower rep ranges (8–10) at an easier effort = faster pace, more total work.

- Higher rep ranges (15–20) at a harder effort = slower pace, fewer rounds.

- Load should allow for consistent movement and quality reps throughout the workout.

Progression Strategy

1. Reduce rest between exercises to increase density by allowing for more reps and sets.

2. Once minimal rest is achieved while maintaining quality movement, extend the time limit and aim to increase intensity or volume while maintaining pace.

Final Considerations

- Volume should be capped to avoid excessive fatigue (e.g., 3–4 MRS per T3, up to 6 sets for T2 squats).

- Adjust exercise selection based on equipment availability. Two to three movements back-to-back can still achieve the goal.

- Don't necessarily avoid, but be mindful of overlapping (e.g., two lower-back-intensive exercises in a row)

- The key is maximizing quality work within the fixed time, not just piling on reps and moving fast mindlessly.

Example Workout B (Fixed Work, Variable Time)

Six Rounds, As Fast As Possible

Giant Set / Circuit

T2a: Bench 10RM@ Working Weight] (Effort Rating) +5 to 8 reps x 4 sets

[Super Set] T3a: Row X-weight x [Target Rep Range] @ (Effort Target) x 4 Max Rep Sets

[Super Set] T3b: Rear Delt Fly X-weight x [Target Rep Range] @ (Effort Target) x 4 Max Rep Sets

[Super Set] T3c: Curls X-weight x [Target Rep Range] @ (Effort Target) x 4 Max Rep Sets

[Super Set] T3d: Jump Rope x [Target Rep Range] @ (Effort Target) x 4 Sets

[Super Set] T3e: Mountain Climbers @Bodyweight x [Target Rep Range] @ (Effort Target) x 4 Sets

Fixed-Work, Variable-Time Conditioning

In this workout, the total work is fixed, and time is the variable. You complete all reps as quickly as possible (while maintaining quality), tracking progress by how much your time improves. Over weeks or months, aim to decrease your time before increasing weight.

Progression Strategy

- Double Progression: Reduce time and increase weight or reps.

- Single Progression: Keep weight the same and focus solely on finishing faster.

- Prioritize density (more work in less time) before adding weight or reps.

Balancing Effort & Recovery

- Set time goals before increasing weight to avoid excessive fatigue.

- If new to conditioning, improve one factor at a time (time before weight or volume).

Cardio & Conditioning Elements

- Fast-paced bodyweight exercises, carries, and jumps enhance conditioning. Include them in your T3.

- Sprinting (rowing, biking, running) can be included, but isn't required for lifting endurance.

- Traditional cardio benefits overall health, but isn't necessary for strength-focused conditioning. It does benefit recovery, especially if the lifter is out of shape.

Final Takeaway

Whether using fixed time and variable work, or fixed work and variable time, the goal is to progressively increase the quality of work you can do in a session while managing recovery.

Rep Max Variations

Skipping or Delaying the Rep Max (RM)

Sometimes, it's beneficial to skip the RM set or perform it last instead of first. While the RM helps gauge progress and develop capacity via VDS, there are valid reasons to modify its placement or omit it entirely.

Why Perform RM Last or Skip It?

- **Technique Focus:** If grinding through an RM set leads to poor form, prioritizing quality volume first can reinforce good technique. This is colloquially known as "greasing the groove." The key factor is that the VDS effort (singles or half-sets) is sufficiently easy. If that is why you're shifting the RM to the last set, all preceding reps should move fast, smooth, and with your best possible form.

  Example: 1 rep x 3 sets +3RM (M). Fourth set as an RM, capped at target effort.

  - This might be the first week of a wave where you're finding new T1 weights that could then be progressed by using the same weight and extending VDS or pushing the RM higher.

- **Building Confidence:** When testing a new T1 weight, doing singles first with a new T1 weight, likewise for half-sets in the T2 (e.g., doubles instead of finding a new 5RM), can make a last set RM attempt more successful as you've "greased the groove" with that weight.

- **Deloading Without Stopping:** Skipping the RM reduces fatigue while still allowing productive work. This is useful when pushing the same weight for weeks and experiencing training fatigue. For example, skipping a 5RM push to a 6RM (or more), instead opting to push half-sets to four reps from three, thereby building more capacity before attempting to push that weight across the T1/T2 bridge.

Example: Skipping RM for a Deload

- **Week 3:** 8RM @ 405 lbs. + 4 reps x 4 sets (Total: 24 reps)

- **Week 4** (Deload): Skip RM + 5 reps x 5 sets (Total: 25 reps)

Despite skipping the RM, total volume increased by pushing the VDS from four to five, improving work capacity without the fatigue associated with the RM set. In the fifth week, the 8RM could be pushed to 9 or 10RM, then aligned with the VDS from Week 4, as shown in the example above.

When to Use This Approach

- Feeling worn down but not ready for a full deload.

- Needing to reduce effort without lowering weight or cutting too many reps.

- Wanting to extend work capacity while managing recovery.

Skipping the RM reduces fatigue while maintaining steady progression, making it a valuable tool for long-term training sustainability.

Skipping the VDS and/or Performing an RM at a Heavier or Lighter Weight than the Volume Sets

The Rep Max (RM) doesn't always need to have its associated Volume Drop Sets (VDS) at the same weight. As a deload option, the VDS can also be skipped. Adjusting volume and intensity ensures rep quality and sustainable progress.

These options can serve different purposes, such as:

- **Deloading Fatigue:** Skipping VDS after such a PR, limiting recovery debt for later workouts. Perhaps that RM PR at a hard effort was absolutely draining, and doing any more volume with that lift seems unreasonable—this is fine! Skip the VDS, whether singles, half-, or three-quarter sets.

- **Testing Strength:** A heavier RM (e.g., a new 5RM PR at a hard effort rating) followed by lighter VDS, comparable to traditional drop sets, while also dropping volume.

  - **Example:** 5RM@315(H)+3x4@275

  - In this case, the 5RM is a PR. But you may not want to skip all the VDS volume, and don't feel ready to do more singles with 315 lbs. (perhaps the set was just that hard!) In this case, you might revert to a weight used as your old 5RM's half-sets in previous weeks. By doing so, you maintain a greater amount of volume while still reaching for those PR weights.

- **Pre-Warmup RM:** Pushing a weight to a higher RM (e.g., turning an 8RM into a 10RM PR) then using a heavier weight to find a separate T2 RM, like a 5RM at a hard effort.

    o **Example:** 10RM@405(H) followed by a 5RM@445(H), or vice versa, working up to the 5RM first followed by the 10RM (this is the traditional drop-set approach).

    o In this case, no VDS is performed because two RM sets were completed, and the volume and effort of this lift in the workout are sufficient. Here, you've identified PRs at the upper end of the T2 and within the T1/T2 bridge. This can also be done with T1 and T2 RM sets.

VDS Flexibility After an RM

- If an RM is unexpectedly harder than planned, reduce the weight for VDS or skip them entirely.

- If an RM is feeling unexpectedly easy, you can take advantage of the opportunity by pushing it for a PR instead of moving to a heavier RM attempt, then keeping the VDS at the originally intended value, thus opening the effort gap.

Example: Target was a 5RM, but the weight was feeling easy and moving well, so you push it to a hard effort 7RM for a PR. Instead of doing half-sets of 3 or 4 reps, which typically follow a 7RM, you keep them at 2 reps, thereby mitigating unplanned fatigue and volume.

Example Adjustments Summary

1. **Easier RM → Heavier VDS**

    o   If your 5 RM PR was much easier than expected, choose a heavier weight for the VDS (whether singles or half-sets).

2. **Lighter RM PR → Continue to Heavy RM**

    o   Push an 8RM to 10RM PR, then proceed cautiously to a 5RM if effort and fatigue allow, or work up to PR attempts of a T1 RM followed by a T2 RM.

3. **RM Too Hard? Adjust VDS**

    o   If a planned 3RM is unexpectedly exhausting, lower the VDS weight or skip singles entirely.

Takeaways

- These choices often happen in the moment, based on how the weights feel.

- Smart adjustments open new progression opportunities while managing fatigue.

- The goal is long-term progression, making heavy weights feel lighter over time.

Skipping the Rep Max to Develop Singles and Volume Drop Sets

I use singles when I want to handle heavy loads without the fatigue of a full T1 RM set. A 3RM PR set can take over a minute from unrack to rerack, leading to significant fatigue. Instead of repeating or finding an RM, I sometimes skip it entirely and perform only singles, allowing for:

- Higher-quality reps at T1 intensities.

- Faster concentric speed compared to fatigued singles and VDS after an RM set.

- Less overall fatigue, making recovery easier, leading to sustained progress.

Example: Managing Fatigue After a 5RM PR

If I set a hard effort 5RM squat PR, my intensity capacity will be low, especially after an accumulation phase. Instead of finding a heavier 5RM the following week, I might:

1. Skip the RM and do only singles using that new 5RM weight. These should be faster than the last reps of an RM, furthering my ability with it. Soon the effort will decrease, allowing me to push it from a 5RM toa 6RM.

2. Skip the RM and gradually increase singles volume, working up to eight total reps over two or three workouts, then going for that RM push.

3. These two options above allow for a return to RM efforts after building confidence and control, likely turning my hard 5RM into an easy 5RM, or even a 6RM attempt due to the accumulation of quality singles.

This approach limits RM exposure while maintaining intensity and volume, ensuring that when I attempt a new RM, it's higher quality and easier. It's beneficial if:

- Confidence under heavy loads is lacking.

- T1 RM sets cause rapid technique breakdown.

- Weekly RM sets cause undue fatigue or mental stress.

Transitioning from Low to High Volume

If I were previously doing 6RM + 3–4 half-sets of 3 reps (~18 total reps), jumping straight to 10RM + 20 VDS reps could be too much next week. This gradual increase in volume prevents over-fatigue while restoring capacity for high-rep efforts.

Applying This to T2 RMs

The same principle applies to T2 VDS after a lower-volume intensification phase. This reduces fatigue while improving work capacity before fully transitioning to higher-rep training.

If stamina is lacking, I might:

- **Week 1**: Skip a 10RM and perform only half-sets (e.g., 5's using an estimated 10RM weight).

- **Week 2:** Turn those half-sets into three-quarter sets (e.g., push those 5's to 7's with that estimated 10RM weight).

- **Week 3:** Go for the 10RM followed by the full amount of VDS via half-sets.

Use this method for 1–2 weeks to transition back to higher-volume training.

Bookend Rep Maxes

Sometimes, an RM set feels too easy. Maybe you underestimated your strength, especially after an accumulation phase. For example, you rack a 5RM only to realize you could have done 8–10 reps and far undershot your effort target. Instead of waiting for next week to correct it, or reattempting a heavier RM (a previously explained option), you can use Bookend RMs:

1. Start with an RM set (e.g., 5RM). It ends up feeling too easy.

2. Perform VDS (singles or half-sets). Limit these to just 2 or 3, making the bookended RM set the third or fourth set performed after the first RM.

3. End with another RM set, pushing the single or half-set until you hit your effort target.

    o Example: 5RM@225(E)+2 reps x 3 sets +7RM@225(H)
    o The 7RM hit the target effort and is the fourth set after the initial 5RM.

4. This can be done with the same weight or with heavier VDS, as previously written.

    o Example: 5RM@225(E)+2 reps x 2 sets +5RM@245(H)
    o The second 5RM was performed with a heavier weight after realizing that the first was too easy and likely too light. The decision was made to limit the VDS to 2x2, reducing

fatigue for the bookended RM attempt at 245, where the target effort was reached.

Bookend RMs are great at developing work capacity and fatigue tolerance, especially when transitioning from an intensification to an accumulation phase. The last RM helps calibrate effort perception and improves next week's weight selection.

When to Use Bookend RMs

- **Effort Calibration:** If you suspect your RM was too easy, a second RM helps dial in your ability at a given weight.

- **Increasing Training Volume:** If a lift (e.g., **bench press**) is stagnating, adding a second RM increases stimulus without excessive fatigue, barring VDS weren't pushed to three-quarter sets and/or extended sets range (5 or 6 sets after the initial RM).

Warning: This is not an every-session strategy. It's highly fatiguing and should be used strategically, when effort assessment or additional volume is needed. If recovery isn't an issue, extend VDS before adding the final RM. This method reveals whether you're undershooting your weights—a good problem to have, since it means you should increase the weight more next week. Remember, if everything feels easy, it is likely too light.

Bottom Line: Bookend RMs refine weight selection, improve effort perception, and can drive progress for stubborn lifts. But be aware of their recovery cost. Use them wisely!

Effort in General Gainz

Effort in General Gainz (GG) measures the perceived difficulty of a set. While Rep Max (RM) sets (T1 & T2) and Max Rep Sets (T3) may sound like they require all-out exertion, they don't necessarily need to be taken to failure. Instead, effort should be rated and applied deliberately to track progress.

For example, if you repeat the same RM as last week, but it feels easier, that's progress. Lower effort in the RM typically allows for more VDS reps, contributing to overall gains in the long run.

Effort isn't just about reps; it also depends on rest periods, tempo, pauses, and bar speed. If an RM feels easy, increase VDS effort by reducing rest, adding pauses, slowing the eccentric, or supersets—this closes the effort gap (the difference in reps between an RM and its VDS).

Effort Ratings

Effort ratings help track progress across all tiers:

- **Easy (E):** 2+ reps in reserve.

- **Moderate (M):** 1 rep in reserve.

- **Hard (H):** No reps left in the tank.

Sets performed without an RM first still require effort ratings for the first and last sets of a session (e.g., 315 lbs., +5 reps x 4 sets, @ Easy on the 1st set to Moderate on the 4th).

In singles-based training, cap volume at the target effort (e.g., 405 lbs., +1 rep x 3-5 sets @ Moderate). If the effort limit is reached before all sets are completed, stop after the 5th set.

Rep Max ≠ Max Effort

An RM isn't just "as many reps as possible." Instead, it factors in technique, bar speed, tempo, pauses, how much volume you want to complete after (via VDS), and rest intervals. Example: If you squat 405x5 at Easy effort, you might pause squat that weight for a Moderate or Hard 1RM.

Rate the RM immediately after the set to avoid second-guessing. If your VDS feels easier than expected, your RM rating might have been too high (you may have rated it hard when it was actually moderate). This system of checks and balances ensures correct effort tracking and helps you gauge your effort accurately.

Effort Gap & Training Progression

The **Effort Gap** is the difference between an RM and its VDS. A wider Effort Gap reduces fatigue from volume sets, improves rep quality across more sets, and enables focused technical work, thereby improving skill. Closing the effort gap develops capacity and strength-endurance by increasing total volume via VDS, reducing rest, or adding intensity techniques (pauses, slow eccentrics, explosive reps).

For example:

- 3RM → Singles = 2-rep gap

- 5RM → Singles = 4-rep gap

- 10RM → Half-sets of 5 = 5-rep gap

Larger effort gaps result in easier VDS. Narrower effort gaps result in more difficult, and thus more fatiguing, VDS. Use the effort gap to apply speed emphasis (CAT), density progression, or a qualitative focus. Alternatively, the effort gap can be closed by increasing volume (e.g., pushing from half-sets to three-quarter sets).

Density & Effort

The best way to make an RM feel easier over time is to increase training density:

1. Shorten rest periods between VDS.

2. Increase how many reps are completed via VDS (more total reps after the RM).

Over time, you will have the ability to push a 5RM to a 10RM and beyond. If follow-up VDS feels too hard, rest longer or reduce the number of reps per VDS. Avoid excessive rest that drastically reduces density.

Adjusting for Effort & Progress

- If the RM was too easy, increase the reps used for VDS (three-quarters rather than half-sets).

- If the RM was too hard, reduce the weight in VDS or reduce the reps per VDS (e.g., performing doubles instead of triples after a 6RM).

- If technique suffers, prioritize pauses, slower eccentrics, or better bar speed over just adding weight, requiring a larger effort gap. Typically, this is done by reducing reps per VDS; however, the traditional drop-set approach can be employed by lowering the weight while keeping the half- and/or three-quarters sets after the RM.

Ultimately, GG thrives on effort regulation, not just intensity and volume. Progress isn't about constantly maxing out; it's about increasing capacity while maintaining quality and intent.

Technical Limit vs. Limit Strength – The Injury Gap

When rating the effort of your lifts, consider these two concepts:

- **Technical limit**: The most weight/reps you can handle while maintaining good technique.

- **Limit strength**: Your absolute max, where technique starts breaking down (e.g., posture shifts, bar path worsens, reps look and move differently as an RM nears completion).

An RM may feel easy if you had more in the tank, but if your technique suffered, it was a hard effort regarding your technical limit. Since technical skill varies by lift, effort must be rated accordingly. A skilled squatter might grind through slow reps with perfect posture, while their bench press could break down quickly, showing no grinding skill on that lift and ending a set due to technical failure rather than muscular exhaustion.

The injury gap is the difference between your technical limit and limit strength. Training with high-quality reps closes this gap, aligns the two, and reduces injury risk. Long-term progress comes from prioritizing movement quality over just lifting heavier.

What is Good Technique?

There's no universal "perfect form." Individual limb proportions create variation—Layne Norton's squat looks different from Tom Platz's, yet both are technically sound because they are consistent and stable.

Good technique means:

- Posture and control remain steady across reps, sets, and sessions.

- The more difficult a set, the more focus is placed on maintaining quality (bar speed, pauses, posture, etc.).

- Maintaining high quality on easy reps should require little effort.

Initially, focusing on the technical limit may feel like a step back if your limit strength is much higher. However, by treating the technical limit as your actual max, you close the injury gap. Eventually, technical and limit strength become indistinguishable—this is mastery. Apply this approach to all movements to train for life with minimal risk of injury and sustained progress.

Progression Planning (Intensity, Volume, Density, Quality)

As explained previously, progression in General Gainz follows four primary forms:

- **Intensity** (weight lifted)

- **Volume** (total reps/sets)

- **Density** (work completed in a given time period)

- **Quality** (consistency and efficiency in the execution of movement)

The first three provide measurable data, while quality is assessed visually and requires honest self-evaluation. Quality underpins all other progressions—poor movement delays progress.

Adaptability in Progression

There is no single "right" way to progress. Clinging to rigid methods leads to stagnation. If sets end in repeated failures, volume becomes unsustainable, rest drags on, and rep quality deteriorates, it's time to adjust.

Progress is maintained through the flexibility of the **Find, Hold, Push, and Extend** principles.

Intensification Progression (Adding Weight)

Definition: The weight lifted relative to 1RM. Increasing weight while maintaining reps. As weight increases, volume naturally declines with individual work capacity.

Example of Intensification Progression

The goal is to increase the weight while maintaining the target reps for as long as possible. When effort becomes too high, reduce reps while continuing to increase weight.

Week-by-Week Progression Example:

- **Weeks 1-3:** 10RM @ 225 +Half-Sets → 235 +Half-Sets → 245 lbs. (Easy) +Half-Sets

- **Weeks 4-5:** 10RM @ 255 (Moderate) +Half-Sets → 265 lbs. (Hard) +Half-Sets

- **Week 6: Rep drop and effort deload** → 8RM @ 275 lbs. (Easy) +Half-Sets

- **Weeks 7-8:** 8RM @ 285 (Moderate) +Half-Sets → 295 lbs. (Hard) +Half-Sets → Volume decreases

- **Week 9: Rep drop and effort deload** → 6RM @ 305 lbs. (Easy) +Half-Sets

- **Week 10-11:** 6RM @ 315 (Easy) +Half-Sets → 5RM @ 325 (Hard) +Half-Sets → Volume drops

- **Week 12:** 5RM @ 335 (Hard), +Singles for Volume Drop Sets

At this stage, a volume decline signals an impending accumulation phase (increasing reps rather than weight). Week 13 begins in the following Accumulation Phase section.

Accumulation Progression (Adding Reps)

Once you reach a lower rep range at your maximum weight, you can hold that weight and increase reps by pushing and extending until a previous 5RM becomes a 10RM. This gradual transition from intensification to accumulation builds sustainable strength.

Definition: Adding reps to a workout by pushing the RM or its half-sets, or by extending those half-sets to their respective limit in the T1 and T2:

- Adding reps (Push). For example: Increasing the RM with a previously used weight and/or making your half-sets fives instead of fours after an 8RM.

- Adding sets while keeping reps the same (Extend).

    o Extending sets: +3 beyond a T1 RM (8 singles after a 5RM).

    o From four half-sets up to six after a T2 RM.

- Increasing total workload across multiple exercises or adding exercises to a workout.

Best done when keeping the weight (intensity) the same from one workout to the next. The key is gradual progression while maintaining rep quality. Adding too much volume too quickly can hinder recovery and performance.

Example Accumulation Progression

This example continues after the previous section's intensification phase, which added 110 pounds over 12 weeks. Once volume reached the minimum desired threshold, an accumulation phase began:

Week 13: 5RM @ 335 lbs. (Moderate) +1 rep x 4 sets

- RM effort dropped from hard to moderate, allowing an extra VDS.

Week 14: 5RM @ 335 lbs. (Easy) +1 rep x 6 sets

- RM felt easier, so VDS increased. Singles extended beyond RM.

Week 15: 6RM @ 335 lbs. (Moderate) +1 rep x 6 sets

- RM increased slightly while maintaining prior VDS.

Week 16: 6RM @ 335 lbs. (Easy) +1 rep x 9 sets

- VDS extended further as the RM effort remained low.

Week 17: 6RM @ 335 lbs. (Easy) +2 reps x 4 sets

- Singles progressed to half-sets, increasing capacity per set.

Week 18: 7RM @ 335 lbs. (Moderate) +3 reps x 4 sets

- RM pushed by one rep, with VDS adjusted accordingly.

Week 19: 7RM @ 335 lbs. (Easy) +3 reps x 6 sets

- RM held, effort reduced, VDS extended to their max.

Week 20: 10RM @ 335 lbs. (Hard) +5 reps x 3 sets

- RM pushed aggressively, reducing VDS due to fatigue.

Week 21-24: Volume continues to build gradually, culminating in a 12RM @ 335 lbs.

Progress Recap

Over 12 weeks (Weeks 13 to 24), RM ability with 335 lbs. doubled from 5RM to 12RM, and total capacity tripled when including VDS data. This sets up another intensification phase, where significant weight can be added while reducing reps, for example, transitioning from 12RM @ 335 to 10RM @ 365 and making your way back towards the T1 by adding weight each week while reducing the target RM as needed.

In this manner, you'll be ebbing and flowing between heavier and lighter phases.

Using a 1RM calculator:

- Week 1: **10RM @ 225 lbs.** → Estimated **1RM @ 300 lbs.**

- Week 24: **12RM @ 335 lbs.** → Estimated **1RM @ 470 lbs.**

Adapting to Your Training

If you're new to General Gainz, use your training data to adjust weight increases and RM targets as you begin using the framework. After several sessions, you'll see trends and know better how to direct your training. You can cycle between intensification and accumulation as needed—some lifters alternate every three weeks to maintain steady progress (and avoid one thing becoming stale). However, such short periodization cycles may not be necessary and may impede long-term progress (hence the above example was extended to 24 weeks).

Lifts will progress at different rates due to individual strengths, preferences, and biomechanics. One lift may be adding weight weekly, while another accumulates volume; that's fine. Outside of competition prep, each lift can follow its own progression based on your ability and recovery.

Density (Work Capacity Progression)

Definition: With Density referring to the amount of work done in a given time, density progression refers to doing more work in less time. This gradually improves your work capacity, allowing you to lift heavier weights for higher rep maxes (RMs) and increase Volume Drop Sets using push or extend actions without compromising your recovery.

Why You Should Care about Work Capacity

Improving your work capacity enhances recovery. The key is increasing training density—doing more reps, then more weight, while holding or reducing rest times as able.

But work capacity isn't just about lifting; it requires cardiovascular conditioning. Incorporate traditional cardio (running, biking, swimming) or gym-based circuits (jump rope, sled, jumping jacks). By sustaining a high heart rate during lifting, you train your muscles to perform for longer and recover faster.

Note that initially, load limits will need to be applied, so you will find T1s much harder to train in this regard (shorter rest periods between singles is tough when an unfit powerlifter, trust me). Therefore, when maintaining a high pace, start with T3s, then add T2s as you cycle in cardio and/or other high-intensity activities.

Work capacity has a specific component. If you aim for high-rep squats, general cardio won't be enough. Your legs must adapt to high-rep squats! Start with isolation exercises (leg curls and extensions) before scaling volume in compound lifts, while keeping rest periods controlled. After several sessions, your legs will be primed for higher-rep squat PRs. The same applies to other muscles if you want high-rep bench PRs; for example, start with high-rep pec flies and triceps pushdowns.

How to Progress Density

- More work (weight/reps/sets) with the same rest periods, or more appropriately, less rest.

- Perform the same weight and volume as a past workout. Complete it faster by reducing rest.

- If you previously lifted 100 lbs. for two reps in 5 seconds and can now do three reps in the same time, you've increased density and work capacity (and also, likely, concentric bar speed. See the section on CAT: Compensatory Acceleration Training).

    o Disclaimer: Truer for compound lifts than isolations. This may not apply to some exercises, like curls, which are better executed with controlled squeezes and stretches rather than lifting as fast as possible regardless of weight.

- Incorporate supersets or circuits

By improving density, you shorten workout duration, freeing up time to add volume to exercises or introduce new ones. If a new RM demands maximum rest periods, hold the weight,

RM, and VDS for the next session, but aim to shorten rest intervals to increase density with that load.

Quarter-Sets

Here's a challenging way to improve density within a session by breaking VDS into smaller chunks:

- After an 8RM, instead of the traditional half-sets (4 reps), perform quarter sets of 2 reps with 30 to 60 seconds rest between each. Time your rest or utilize an EMOM-style timer.

- Since these are quarter sets, double the VDS count to hit the usual T2 volume—8 to 12 doubles after the 8RM.

Progressing Quarter-Set Density

- **Time your exercises** (from the RM to the last double) and aim to complete them faster next session. Fifteen seconds between quarter sets is moving fast.

- **Increase reps per set** (e.g., turn doubles into triples) while keeping the total duration the same.

Quality (Mastering Lifts. Beyond the Numbers)

Progress isn't just about adding weight or volume or reducing rest. Also consider refining lift quality. While speed is a quality that may have data too, other aspects require honest self-assessment.

Improving Lift Quality

- **Posture & Consistency**: Maintain proper positioning rep after rep.

- **Rhythm & Coordination**: Smooth, controlled movement patterns.

- **Balance & Control**: Stability and precision under a load.

- **Efficiency & Fluidity**: Minimize wasted effort and jerky transitions.

If your reps at a given weight are inconsistent or sloppy, prioritize quality before increasing load or volume. A new movement should emphasize rep rhythm, coordination, and positional stability before progressing.

The closer you push toward limit strength, the more quality breaks down—especially in long sets. A 20RM squat might look great for the first 15 reps, but fatigue will test your posture, rhythm, and control in the final five reps.

The stronger and more skilled you are, the longer quality holds up under heavy loads.

Mastering a Weight

Getting stronger requires lifting heavier. Improving execution is part of that. Mastering a weight means:

- Better tempo control, posture, and rep consistency.

- Lifting the same weight faster through compensatory acceleration.

- Reducing rest periods while maintaining output.

During accumulation phases, holding a weight for multiple sessions enhances quality. Performing singles after a T1 RM allows precise tracking of bar speed and control. If a weight always feels heavy, train it frequently, focusing on execution rather than just adding plates to try to beat it through intensification. Instead, go for quality (speed foremost). If you're using the same weight for consecutive sessions and it starts feeling lighter: congratulations, you're stronger.

Tracking and Refining Quality

Strength progression often gets reduced to numbers, but video analysis helps assess unseen improvements:

- If a rep is slow, identify why (poor tension, eccentric control, lack of focus, fatigue, etc.).

- Review lifts between sets to pinpoint errors and refine execution.

- Strive for consistent position, speed, and control across reps and sets.

Lifters obsessed with "optimal" numbers often overlook quality. Progress can be observed through data and with the naked eye. Spreadsheets mask things that should be addressed, but they make it easy to collect information. Many of us hoard data needlessly. Imagine all those spreadsheets like stacks of junk cluttering your house, and how awful it must be to live in such a house. Now, consider that aspect as one reason why you've not enjoyed training… perhaps you've been overthinking and overplanning: hoarding junk you'd live better without. Ditch some data and instead observe quality.

Recovery

Recovery doesn't mean inactivity. If training leaves you immobilized for days, you need more movement, not less. Recovery is dictated by work capacity, not always opting for doing less.

Increase recovery ability by staying active. GPP work (e.g., sled pushes, carries, jump rope) or manual labor (e.g., shoveling, digging) builds resilience.

If you dislike weights, walk, run, or bike. Move often and vigorously, and don't make any excuses; find a way to do it.

Three Pillars of Recovery

1. Nutrition & Hydration

- **Calories**: Eat enough to fuel training. ± 250 calories from maintenance is a good guideline for bulking or cutting without compromising energy.

- **Protein**: Aim for 0.7–1.0g per pound of body weight to maintain or build muscle. Some argue that more is better. How much more is helpful is debatable.

- **Hydration**: Water alone isn't enough. Electrolytes matter. Even 1% dehydration impairs performance; a 2.5% loss can drop high-intensity output by 45%. Carry a water bottle, drink consistently, and be mindful of your intake after 4 PM to avoid disrupting sleep. The importance of proper hydration cannot be understated.

2. Sleep

- **Sleep = performance.** Six hours may keep you functional, but your performance will be far from your best. Aim for 7–8 hours of sleep to support gains in size, strength, and endurance.

- **Improve sleep hygiene**: A set bedtime, use a cooling mattress, put on white noise, use a humidifier, nasal strips, and meditation. Find what helps and use it consistently.

- **Napping**: Add short naps when able! These help with day-to-day lethargy, reducing overall fatigue and exhaustion, which can negatively impact your training.

3. De-stressing

- **Chronic stress kills recovery.** Cut out needless stressors. Limit toxic interactions, avoid stressful commutes, and unplug from constant news and social media.

- **Stress management**: Reading, philosophy (e.g., stoicism), prayer, and meditation help offset unavoidable stress.

- **Training is stress application, not stress relief.** While it may feel like an escape, it still taxes your system. Recover actively, not passively.

Resting is more than merely spending time out of the gym doing nothing. It's training smarter, recovering better, and living better. Replace mindless "recovery" on the couch with proactive movement, good habits, and stress management.

Don't rest lazily, thinking it means you're recovering. Recover by being modestly active.

Rest Days

For me, training daily has led to better workout management, preventing me from overdoing it in a single session, week, or month. When I took rest days, I justified excessive training by thinking, "I'll recover this weekend" or "I have a vacation next week, so I'll go hard now." This mindset changed when I committed to training every day.

Knowing I will train tomorrow helps me regulate my effort accurately. General Gainz supports high-frequency training, but it doesn't require it. Your plan, whether you train three, four, five, six, or seven days a week, or even two-a-days, should align with your schedule and recovery capacity. Take rest days as needed or train daily if you prefer.

Because GG is intuitive and flexible, I've been able to train consistently without rest days, avoiding both overtraining and undertraining. Daily feedback from my workouts allows me to adjust my training volume and intensity as needed. As a result, I've achieved both specific goals, such as PRs in various barbell lifts and muscle growth in my arms and shoulders, and general goals, such as getting bigger and fitter overall. These can be measured using metrics such as scale weight, tape measurements, or workouts that test strength and stamina.

The belief that "progress is made outside the gym" is a platitude. Many who have run GG, including myself, have found that structured daily training can work without traditional rest days—if recovery habits (nutrition, hydration, sleep, and stress management) are prioritized. If rest days encourage you to train recklessly or neglect good recovery habits, they may slow your progress.

That said, I'm not against rest days. If you need them for health, injury, or lifestyle reasons, take them. But if you want to train daily, you can. You should be physically active every day in some form, whether that's lifting, walking, swimming, martial arts, or even frisbee golf. Start light, build volume and intensity gradually, and you'll improve strength, size, and stamina without recovery debt.

I haven't had a rest day in over six years (just after developing GG), nor am I the first to thrive with daily training. But GG makes it easy. Rest days are not forbidden. They're one variable of a multi-variable process. More frequent training fosters consistency, and consistency drives progress. Let this encourage you to practice daily physicality.

Progression Models & Pre-Made Programs

This section offers training programs designed as templates for you to build your own plans. Each program follows a progression that utilizes the four actions: find, hold, push, and extend. If you're unsure about these at any point, refer to the "Four Actions" section for clarification.

Use these programs as inspiration. Tailor them to your goals, abilities, and limitations by changing exercises or adjusting weight and reps based on your training data. Remember, these programs aren't necessarily meant to be followed exactly as written; customize them to make your training personal. Owning your progression makes it more rewarding and effective.

Example Weekly Schedules

Your lifting schedule will depend on how many days per week you can train.

- **2-3 days/week:** Full-body workouts are recommended.

- **4 days/week:** A split between upper and lower body allows for more recovery and more demanding sessions.

- **5+ days/week:** Splits based on either lifts (for strength) or muscle groups (for aesthetics). This allows for higher frequency, enabling you to hone a lift or give more attention to a lagging muscle group.

With more frequent training, you can include more exercises or increase intensity/volume. For example, powerlifters may squat and bench multiple times a week and deadlift twice. General training enthusiasts may want more variety across all tiers.

Keep in mind that as training frequency increases, you'll be able to handle more total volume, but only after having acclimated. A seven-day plan will require lower volume per session at first. As the weeks progress, each workout will allow you to do a little more, such as adding exercises or increasing intensity and/or volume more aggressively.

For beginners, start with fewer exercises and lighter progressions. New lifters might begin with three or four exercises per workout rather than five. Adjust as needed to suit your level.

Be intentional with any volume or intensity increases. Stray from the program when needed.

Example Schedules

Be aware that these example schedules may not be perfectly balanced for your needs and should be treated only as a starting point. Feel free to adjust exercises to fit your goals, abilities, and preferences.

Two Days Per Week

Day 1
T1 Squat
T1 Bench
T2 Romanian Deadlift
T3a Lat Pull Down
T3b Seated DB Press
T3c Leg Curls
T3d Leg Extensions

Day 2
T1 Press
T1 Deadlift
T2 Incline Bench
T3a Leg Press
T3b Barbell Row
T3c Overhead Triceps Extension
T3d Biceps Curl

Three Days Per Week

Day 1
T1 Squat
T2 Press
T3a Barbell Row
T3b Calf Raise
T3c Decline Sit-Up
T3d Cable Curl

Day 2
T1 Bench
T1 Front Squat
T2 Lat Pull Down
T3a Seated DB Press
T3b Rear Delt Fly
T3c Overhead Triceps Extension

Day 3
T1 Deadlift
T1 Incline Bench
T2 Underhand Cable Row
T3a DB Bench
T3b Leg Curl
T3c Leg Extension

Four Days Per Week

Day 1
T1 Squat
T2 Press
T3a Pull-Ups
T3b Side Crunch
T3c Decline Sit-Up
T3d Ab Straps

Day 2
T1 Bench
T1 Sumo Deadlift
T2 Underhand Barbell Row
T3a Strict Curl
T3b Overhead Triceps Extension
T3c Rear Delt Fly

Day 3
T1 Press
T2 Front Squat
T3a Incline DB Bench
T3b Lat Pull Down
T3c Cable Row
T3d DB Shrug

Day 4
T1 Deadlift
T1 Close-Grip Bench
T2 Leg Press
T3a Leg Curl
T3b Leg Extension
T3c Cable Triceps Push Down

Five Days Per Week

Day 1
T1 Squat
T2 Lunges
T3a Side Crunch
T3b Leg Lifts
T3c Decline Sit Ups

Day 2
T1 Bench
T2 Press
T3a Incline DB Bench
T3b Pec Fly
T3c Overhead Triceps Extension

Day 3
T1 Deadlift
T2 Romanian Deadlift
T3a Pull-Ups
T3b Cable Row
T3c Strict Curl

Day 4
T1 Press
T2 Incline Bench
T3a DB Bench
T3b Lateral Raise
T3c Cable Triceps Push Down

Day 5
T1 Power Clean
T2 Front Squat
T3a 45-Degree Hyper
T3b Reverse Hyper
T3c Cable Twist

Six Days Per Week

Day 1
T1 Squat
T2 Lunges
T3a Side Crunch
T3b Leg Lifts
T3c Decline Sit Ups

Day 2
T1 Bench
T2 Press
T3a Incline DB Bench
T3b Pec Fly
T3c Overhead Triceps Extension

Day 3
T1 Deadlift
T2 Romanian Deadlift
T3a Pull-Ups
T3b Cable Row
T3c Strict Curl

Day 4
T1 Press
T2 Incline Bench
T3a DB Bench
T3b Lateral Raise
T3c Cable Triceps Push Down

Day 5
T1 Power Clean
T2 Front Squat
T3a 45-Degree Hyper
T3b Reverse Hyper
T3c Cable Twist

Day 6
T1 Push Press
T2 Close Grip Bench
T3a Dips
T3b Seated DB Shoulder Press
T3c EZ Bar Curl

Note: I don't program a seventh training day. Though I train daily, I cycle through three-, four-, and six-day schedules, with workouts not fixed to a calendar day. Adjust per your needs.

Powerlifting Considerations

If training for powerlifting, your T1 lifts should be competition-specific (squat, bench, deadlift), while T2 lifts should be close variations (pause or front squat, close-grip bench, Romanian deadlift). Keep T2 rep maxes around 5RM-6RM to bridge strength gains. Adjust T3 work based on T1 and T2 performance, ensuring it supports rather than interferes with your main lifts.

Bodybuilding Considerations

For aesthetic goals, minimize T1 work, especially heavy singles. Occasional 3RM-5RM lifts are fine, but prioritize T2 and T3 with higher volume. Use accumulation models (progressing via added reps and sets) and experiment with supersets—either complementary (rear delt fly + lat pulldown) or antagonistic (pec fly + lat pulldown).

For a deeper dive into my bodybuilding experience with the GG framework, check out my blog: General Gainz Body Building.

GG Linear Progression (GGLP)

GGLP follows two primary progression models: **Intensification** (adding weight) and **Accumulation** (adding reps). Other factors, such as reducing rest, can play a role but aren't the primary focus.

Though you may sometimes progress in both weight and reps simultaneously, GGLP typically prioritizes one at a time. Commit to a minimum of **3–6 weeks** of either intensification or accumulation before switching. This approach benefits both beginners and experienced lifters returning to linear progression. While later programs in GG incorporate GGLP elements, the base form remains distinct and effective for all levels.

GGLP Intensification (GGLPI)

This method progresses by adding weight each week while maintaining volume limits based on your RM. Reps decrease naturally as effort increases due to the weekly weight increases.

Example Progression:

- **Week 1:** 5RM @ 135 lbs. (Easy) + 3 reps × 4–6 sets

- **Week 2:** 5RM @ 140 lbs. (Easy) + 3 reps × 4–6 sets

- **Week 3:** 5RM @ 145 lbs. (Moderate) + 3 reps × 4–6 sets

- **Week 4:** 5RM @ 150 lbs. (Moderate) + 2 reps × 4–6 sets

- **Week 5:** 5RM @ 155 lbs. (Moderate) + 2 reps × 4–6 sets

- **Week 6:** 5RM @ 160 lbs. (Hard) + 1 rep × 5–8 sets

Key Points

- Volume is held as long as possible while weight increases.

- Reps per VDS decrease as effort rises. Total volume can be kept from reducing too quickly by extending the VDS to its limit.

- By week 6, singles maintain rep quality, and total volume approaches the T1 limit (+3 beyond the RM). Subsequent weeks may continue to add weight and reduce singles volume as needed.

- This process moves an RM from T2 (VDS are half- and three-quarter sets) to T1 (VDS are singles) by gradually increasing effort at a fixed rep target.

GGLP Accumulation (GGLPA)

This method progresses by adding reps to the same weight each week, either by increasing the RM, VDS reps, or number of VDS completed.

Example Progression

- **Week 1:** 5RM @ 135 lbs. (Easy) + 3 reps × 4–6 sets

- **Week 2:** 6RM @ 135 lbs. (Easy) + 3 reps × 4–6 sets

- **Week 3:** 7RM @ 135 lbs. (Moderate) + 3 reps × 4–6 sets

- **Week 4:** 7RM @ 135 lbs. (Easy) + 4 reps × 4–6 sets

- **Week 5:** 8RM @ 135 lbs. (Moderate) + 4 reps × 4–6 sets

- **Week 6:** 9RM @ 135 lbs. (Hard) + 5 reps × 4–6 sets

Key Points

- Reps increase weekly, either to the RM or to the VDS.

- Should an RM be the same week to week, but it was easier, increase VDS reps as is the case in the third and fourth weeks above (from 3s to 4s).

- Higher RMs bring the movement closer to the T3 range, making VDS feel easier due to the Effort Gap. After a hard 9RM, sets of five reps may move well and feel easy. If so, consider pushing VDS from half to three-quarters in Week 7, which may result in a moderate 9RM effort. This would mirror the action taken with the repeated 7RM in weeks three and four.

Both methods, intensification and accumulation, can be extended, depending on individual response. Progress occurs so long as weight or reps are added each week. Flow between these methods as fit.

Some lifts may continue an intensification progression longer than accumulation; this is fine. Unless you're using a fixed progression pattern, this "natural" progression is acceptable and encouraged. When training within the GG framework but outside a fixed progression model, note that not every lift needs to progress using the same method or at the same rate.

GG Wave LP (Waves of Intensification and Accumulation)

GG Wave LP structures training cycles by alternating **intensification** (progressing load at a fixed rep max – Find) and **accumulation** (increasing volume at a stable load – Push and/or "Extend). These waves can be preplanned in 3- or 4-week cycles or adjusted dynamically based on performance.

Example Progression

Fixed 6-Week Cycle (No T1 Lift. A higher volume "Bodybuilding" approach)

- **Intensification Phase**

    - **Week 1:** Find 5RM (easy effort). Add weight next week.

    - **Week 2:** Find 5RM (easy to moderate effort). Add weight next week.

    - **Week 3:** Find 5RM (moderate to hard effort).

- **Accumulation Phase**

    - **Week 4:** Hold 5RM weight, effort should decrease. Increase VDS reps (e.g., turning doubles into triples and/or attempting a bookend RM set).

    - **Week 5:** Push weight to 6RM if volume was maximized last week. Follow with triples or doubles based on effort.

o **Week 6:** Push to 7RM+ if volume was maximized at 6RM. Follow with half-sets (e.g., triples after a hard 7RM).

Bench Press (T2a)

	RM	Weight	Effort	Follow-Up Reps	Sets
Week 1	5	295	E	3	6
Week 2	5	300	E	3	5
Week 3	5	305	M	2	6
Week 4	5	305	E	3	5
Week 5	6	305	H	3	6
Week 6	7	305	H	3	4

In this example, a bridge weight has been pushed deeper into the T2 range. Consider that, before this wave, the lifter may have lifted 295 pounds for several weeks, pushing it from a 3RM to a 5RM, with fully extended half-sets afterward.

Key Points

- **VDS Adjustments**: Adjust sets and reps based on effort. For example, if a 5RM was easy, VDS may stay at triples, but if it was moderate, doubles allow for better fatigue management.

- **Effort Gaps**: Larger rep drops (e.g., from 5RM to doubles) allow more VDS due to reduced fatigue, offering the ability to extend sets up to six.

- **Autoregulation**: If a weight increase reduces RM performance (e.g., a 5RM turns into a hard 4RM), adjust VDS accordingly (e.g., shifting from doubles to singles for better quality reps throughout the VDS). Extend the VDS as able, based on rep quality.

Adding a Second Lift (T2 Example)

A secondary lift follows a similar cycle but at a different intensity range.

- **Example: Squat (T2)**

    o   Week 1: Start at an 8RM (light T2).

    o   Week 2: Add weight (Find) to the 8RM, hold volume based on effort increases.

    o   Week 3: Repeat Week 2.

    o   Week 4-6: Hold weight and increase RM, or reps per VDS or total VDS, adjusting based on effort.

        ▪   Push/Extend T2 half-sets to three-quarter sets and/or perform up to six of these sets after the RM.

        ▪   When VDS has reached its limit, push the RM higher.

This approach ensures progression while balancing fatigue and volume across multiple lifts.

In the above progression example, an 8RM target of 425 lbs. is held for three weeks. As the weeks progress, the effort gradually declines. As a result of this decrease in effort, the total volume of the VDS increases. The "4,3" under the follow-up column means that the lifter started with fours but moved to threes as rep quality declined across the five sets completed. Over the next two weeks, the VDS value increased to 4, then to 5 as the 8RM got easier.

Accessory Progression Model

T3 exercises follow a structured progression within intensification or accumulation phases.

Intensification (Increasing Load, Decreasing Reps)

- **Week 1:** Find weight in the range of 12-15 reps, 3-4 sets (easy effort).

- **Week 2:** Add Weight, 10-12 reps, 3-4 sets (moderate effort).

Squat (T2b)

	RM	Weight	Effort	Follow-Up Reps	Sets
Week 1	8	405	E	4	6
Week 2	8	415	E	4,3	6
Week 3	8	425	M	4,3	5
Week 4	8	425	M	4	6
Week 5	8	425	E	5	5
Week 6	10	425	H	5	4

- **Week 3:** Add Weight, 8-10 reps, 2-3 sets (hard effort).

Seated DB Press (T3a)
Lat Pull Down (T3b)
Overhead Cable Triceps Extension (T3c)
Cable Biceps Curl (T3d)

	Target Rep Range	Weight	Target Effort	# of Sets
Week 1	12 to 15	?	E	3 to 4
Week 2	10 to 12	?	M	3 to 4
Week 3	8 to 10	?	H	2 to 3
Week 4	8 to 10	?	M	3 to 4
Week 5	10 to 12	?	M	3 to 4
Week 6	12 to 15	?	H	2 to 3

Accumulation (Holding Load, Increasing Reps)

- **Week 4:** Same Weight, 8-10 reps, 3-4 sets (effort should be easier than last week).

- **Week 5:** Same weight, 10-12 reps, 3-4 sets (moderate effort).

- **Week 6:** Same weight, 12-15 reps, 2-3 sets (hard effort).

Summary

Intensification = Load Progression (heavier weights, fewer reps, load increases effort).

Accumulation = Volume Progression (same weight, more reps, volume increases effort).

T3 Exercises: Can flow between both intensification and accumulation. Beginners or those needing more work capacity can benefit from accumulation phases.

Autoregulation: Adjust RM target and VDS based on effort, fatigue, and performance trends.

This structured approach allows continuous progression while managing recovery and training quality.

If you need to build work capacity, prioritize T3 accumulation cycles. These cycles not only improve endurance but also provide more practice with a variety of exercises.

Use the GG Wave LP framework to structure your workouts based on your schedule and goals. Whether training two to three times per week with full-body sessions or six times per week with a split routine, apply the progression model accordingly.

Your actual progression will vary based on performance data and key actions (find, hold, push, extend). Consider it as inspiration rather than a strict template.

Wave LP is open-ended. Later programs build on this concept with fixed-length progression models. There are many ways to structure workouts in this fashion, allowing each lift to progress through its own wave independently (not all lifts have to progress in the same way).

The following is the second example, which includes a T1 lift (RM followed by singles) and two T2 lifts at opposite ends of the T2 RM range. This would be more suitable for a powerlifter, before a peaking wave.

The T3 follows a repeating intensification cycle. This T3 approach is simple, and I've found it beneficial for limiting fatigue. One reason is the ability to cycle in new lifts with each successive wave. This keeps the session interesting, challenging, and fun.

General Gainz - Wave LP

Example progression - Example workout

Deadlift (T1)

	RM	Weight	Effort	Follow-Up Reps	Sets
Week 1	3	500	E	1	6
Week 2	3	510	M	1	5
Week 3	3	520	H	1	3
Week 4	3	520	M	1	4
Week 5	3	520	M	1	6
Week 6	4	520	M	1	7

Front Squat (T2a)

	RM	Weight	Effort	Follow-Up Reps	Sets
Week 1	5	305	E	3	6
Week 2	5	315	E	3,2	6
Week 3	5	325	M	2	6
Week 4	6	325	H	2	6
Week 5	6	325	M	3,2	6
Week 6	7	325	H	3	5

Strict Barbell Row (T2b)

	RM	Weight	Effort	Follow-Up Reps	Sets
Week 1	8	225	E	4	6
Week 2	8	235	M	4	5
Week 3	8	245	H	4	4
Week 4	8	245	M	4	6
Week 5	9	245	H	5	5
Week 6	10	245	H	5	4

Leg Press (T3a)

45-Degree Hyper Extension (T3b)

Quadriceps Extension (T3c)

Hamstring Curl (T3d)

	Target Rep Range	Weight	Target Effort	# of Sets
Week 1	12 to 15	?	E	3 to 4
Week 2	10 to 12	?	M	3 to 4
Week 3	8 to 10	?	H	2 to 3
Week 4	8 to 10	?	M	3 to 4
Week 5	10 to 12	?	M	3 to 4
Week 6	12 to 15	?	H	2 to 3

Fixed Length Programs

Riptide

Riptide is an 8-week, adaptable program that will challenge your limits, utilizing a unique blend of rep-max cycling. By limiting very heavy T1 work, Riptide biases hypertrophy and muscular endurance.

Whether you prefer a full-body approach or a split (upper/lower or movement-based), Riptide can fit into your personal schedule.

Be familiar with the four actions (find/hold/push/extend) to further personalize this progression to your ability, recovery, and goals.

T1 Maximal Strength

Each workout begins with a single exercise aimed at maximal strength. The progression alternates between finding heavy rep maxes in odd weeks (e.g., Week 1: 5RM, Week 3: 3RM) and pushing those rep maxes in even weeks (e.g., Week 2: hitting 6 reps with last week's 5RM). VDS are singles in odd weeks. Half-sets on even weeks after an RM push. Adjust those per previous guidance based on the RM effort. As your maximal strength increases, so does your ability to push the weights for more reps.

T2 Strength Endurance

Building on the foundational strength of T1, T2 utilizes moderate weights (10RM down to 5RM) to increase volume and muscular endurance. The same alternating progression applies here: max reps at a specific weight in odd weeks, and push those weights to higher RMs in even weeks. The total number of sets and reps will vary based on effort levels and fatigue, ensuring optimal muscle stimulus.

T3 Hypertrophy

T3 is designed to build muscular endurance, focusing on higher reps: start with lighter, easy-effort sets of 15-20 reps, then progress to harder, high-effort sets of 8-10 reps.

Key Features:

Flexibility: Full-body or split training, depending on your schedule and preference.

Lighter T1 Progression: Less maximal strength emphasis. Greater hypertrophy emphasis due to the total volume not being limited by weekly T1 singles.

Adaptive Structure: Deliberate effort cycles to ensure consistent recovery and growth.

The example workout progression shows one day across eight weeks. This session is an upper-body workout. Your Riptide schedule can be an upper/lower split like the example, or a movement or body-part split.

If you are a powerlifter, you can implement higher lift frequency by utilizing full-body sessions. That depends on your capacity. Use the previous Example Schedules section as inspiration.

Consider running Riptide in reverse:

Undertow

Begin with week 7's 2RM, push that weight to a higher RM in Week 8. Then find a 4RM in week 5, and push that weight to a higher RM the following week. Then find your 3RM and push that for a higher RM the week after. Then the 5RM attempt followed the next week by pushing that to a higher RM.

The paragraph above describes working backward through the Riptide progression. The key factor is still performing the Find RM weeks before the Push RM weeks. If following Riptide with Undertow, the RM attempts should be heavier than those found when running Riptide.

Riptide & Undertow (GG R&T) can work together in alternating fashion. I encourage you to rotate your T1 lift into your T2 and vice versa.

As you see, the wave theme persists. This is because I've found such progression best (either intensification or accumulation, based on lifter needs) due to its fluidity and seemingly endless repeatability.

Many of the key features of GG R&T are also present in the following programs, though uniquely so.

General Gainz - Riptide (& Undertow)

Example Workout

Bench Press (T1)   Follow-Up

	RM	Weight	Effort	Reps	Sets
Week 1	5	Find (?)	E	2 or 3	4 to 6
Week 2	Push RM	Hold Wk1	H	1/2 of RM	4 to 6
Week 3	3	Find (?)	M	1	3 to 6
Week 4	Push RM	Hold Wk3	H	1	If RM < 5, singles.
					Match RM min.
					+3 over RM max.
				1/2 of RM	If RM > 5, 1/2 sets.
					4 sets min. 6 max.
Week 5	4	Find (?)	E	1	4 to 7
Week 6	Push RM	Hold Wk5	H	1	If RM < 5, singles.
					Match RM min.
					+3 over RM max.
				1/2 of RM	If RM > 5, 1/2 sets.
					4 sets min. 6 max.
Week 7	2	Find (?)	M	1	1 to 2
Week 8	Push RM	Hold Wk7	H	Skip	Skip
					No additional sets this week.

Effort ratings indicate both RM target effort and when to stop performing singles. Goal is: sets range + target effort. Example: When effort is M, stop when only one more single can be completed (then a hard effort). If the limit of singles is completed at an easier effort, then good, so long as they moved fast and rest times were minded.

Strict Press (T2)   Follow-Up

	RM	Weight	Effort	Reps	Sets
Week 1	10	Find (?)	E	5	4 to 6
Week 2	Push RM	Hold Wk1	H	1/2 of RM	4 to 6
Week 3	6	Find (?)	M	3	4 to 6
Week 4	Push RM	Hold Wk3	H	1/2 of RM	4 to 6
Week 5	8	Find (?)	E	4	4 to 6
Week 6	Push RM	Hold Wk5	H	1/2 of RM	4 to 6
Week 7	5	Find (?)	M	2	4 to 6
Week 8	Push RM	Hold Wk7	H	1/2 of RM	4 to 6

Lat Pull Down (T3a)

Cable Row (T3b)

Cable Curl (T3c)

Rear Delt Fly (T3d)

	Target Rep Range	Weight	Target Effort	# of Sets
Week 1	15 to 20	?	E	3 to 4
Week 2	12 to 15	?	E	3 to 4
Week 3	10 to 12	?	M	3 to 4
Week 4	8 to 10	?	H	2 to 3
Week 5	15 to 20	?	E	3 to 4
Week 6	12 to 15	?	E	3 to 4
Week 7	10 to 12	?	M	3 to 4
Week 8	8 to 10	?	H	2 to 3

Iron Tides

Iron Tides is built on this same principle: a training progression that moves in measured cycles, building strength, size, and stamina. This is not a program of brute force or reckless intensity. It is a calculated approach that ebbs and flows, allowing lifters to push further without breaking, to advance without losing their footing.

T1 Maximal Strength

One movement, heavy and deliberate, following a repeating 3-week cycle. The weight remains constant, while effort and volume slowly increase. Develop singles for two weeks by adding to them. Perform two to three singles in the first week, followed by four to six singles in the second. In the third week, find an RM with that same weight, followed by no VDS after this RM set.

Waves gather before surging.

T2 Strength Endurance

Two exercises, each with its own 6-week cycle. These swells rise higher, layering intensity with volume and effort. T2a progressing from 10RM to 6RM. T2b does the same, but from 12RM to 8RM. The waves grow higher each week.

T3 Hypertrophy

Four exercises, flowing in their own 3-week progression from 15 to 6 reps per set. The watery deep where Leviathan lifts, and lifters grow.

General Gainz - Iron Tides

Example Workout

Press (T1)

	RM	Weight	Effort	Follow-Up Reps	Sets
Week 1	Skip	?	E	1	2 to 3
Week 2	Skip	Hold	M	1	4 to 6
Week 3	Find RM	Hold	H	Skip	Skip

Repeat this wave. Add weight when repeating. If weight cannot be added, work on being more explosive with the same weight or reducing rest between sets.

Effort ratings indicate both RM target effort and when to stop performing singles. Goal is: sets range + target effort. Example: When effort is M, stop when only one more single can be completed. If the limit of singles is completed at an easier effort, then good, so long as they moved fast and rest times were maintained.

Incline Bench (T2a)

	RM	Weight	Effort	Follow-Up Reps	Sets
Week 1	10	?	E	5	4 to 6
Week 2	Push RM	Hold	M	1/2 of RM	3 to 4
Week 3	8	?	E	4	4 to 6
Week 4	Push RM	Hold	M	1/2 of RM	3 to 4
Week 5	6	?	M	3	4 to 6
Week 6	Push RM	Hold	H	1/2 of RM	3 to 4

Bench (T2b)

	RM	Weight	Effort	Follow-Up Reps	Sets
Week 1	12	?	E	6	4 to 6
Week 2	Push RM	Hold	M	1/2 of RM	3 to 4
Week 3	10	?	E	5	4 to 6
Week 4	Push RM	Hold	M	1/2 of RM	3 to 4
Week 5	8	?	M	4	4 to 6
Week 6	Push RM	Hold	H	1/2 of RM	3 to 4

T3a Overhead Cable Triceps Extension
T3b 1-Arm Cable Lateral Raise
T3c Pec Fly
T3d Rear Delt Fly

	Target Rep Range	Weight	Target Effort	# of Sets
Week 1	12 to 15	?	M	3 to 4
Week 2	10 to 12	?	M	3 to 4
Week 3	8 to 10	?	H	1 to 2
Week 4	10 to 12	?	M	3 to 4
Week 5	8 to 10	?	M	3 to 4
Week 6	6 to 8	?	H	1 to 2

Abyssal Wake

Abyssal Wake is a 12-week program. Its structure combines T1 maximal-strength building, T2 volume development, and longer T3 intensification cycles.

Abyssal Wake has its own unique progression waves.

T1 Maximal Strength

T1 focuses on heavier rep-maxes and singles. Each workout begins with one exercise, starting at 5RM in week one and progressing to singles. The number of singles depends on the RM's effort. Maximize singles while minding rep quality (CAT).

Weeks 5 and 6 introduce an inversion in the wave, where you'll perform singles first with a last set RM. Weeks in which the last set is the RM are the only hard-effort weeks. Push yourself in these weeks, use them to hone your effort gauge.

Weeks 7 through 12 cycle through the heavier 3RM, 2RM, and Singles with a last set RM.

T2 Strength Endurance

T2 starts at the lighter end of its range, progressing to the heavier end: 10RM through 5RM. The first six weeks add weight, working towards heavier RM sets.

In weeks 7-12, push those RMs higher, i.e., making the week one 10RM a 12RM in week seven.

This combination of continued overload with added volume sets promotes sustained hypertrophy and strength progression. Review the Four Actions section to familiarize yourself with progression options should the RM push efforts not go according to plan in the second half of the program, i.e., if the RM push is unsuccessful, shift focus to increasing the volume by pushing half-sets to three-quarter sets.

T3 Hypertrophy

Four exercises per workout. Progressively reduce reps while increasing weight over the course of the 12 weeks. Effort increases weekly, E/M/H, allowing for weight increases while staying in the target rep range.

Wave A: 15-20 reps per set

Wave B: 12-15 reps, focusing on maintaining quality with slightly heavier loads.

Wave C: 10-12, going heavier still while maintaining quality.

Wave D: 8-10 per set, even heavier, with quality reps.

General Gainz - Abyssal Wake

Example Workout

Squat (T1)

	RM	Weight	Effort	Follow-Up Reps	Sets
Week 1	5	?	E	1	5 Min./8 max.
Week 2	4	?	E	1	4 Min./7 max.
Week 3	3	?	M	1	3 Min./6 max.
Week 4	2	?	M	1	1 to 2
Week 5	Last Set RM	?	H	1	3 singles, 4th set RM.
Week 6	Last Set RM	?	H	1	2 singles, 3rd set RM.
Week 7	3	?	M	1	3 Min./6 max.
Week 8	2	?	M	1	1 to 2
Week 9	Last Set RM	?	H	1	3 singles, 4th set RM.
Week 10	3	?	M	1	3 Min./6 max.
Week 11	2	?	M	1	1 to 2
Week 12	Last Set RM	?	H	1	2 singles, 3rd set RM.

Singles in Wk5 should be heavier than 2RM in Wk4.

Wk6 likewise to Wk5. Wk9 & Wk12 respectively.

Romanian Deadlift (T2)

	RM	Weight	Effort	Follow-Up Reps	Sets
Week 1	10	?	E	5	4 to 6
Week 2	9	?	M	4 or 5	4 to 6
Week 3	8	?	H	4	4 to 6
Week 4	7	?	E	3 or 4	4 to 6
Week 5	6	?	M	3	4 to 6
Week 6	5	?	H	2 or 3	4 to 6
Week 7	Push	Wk1	E	1/2 of RM	4 to 6
Week 8	Push	Wk2	M	1/2 of RM	4 to 6
Week 9	Push	Wk3	H	1/2 of RM	4 to 6
Week 10	Push	Wk4	E	1/2 of RM	4 to 6
Week 11	Push	Wk5	M	1/2 of RM	4 to 6
Week 12	Push	Wk6	H	1/2 of RM	4 to 6

T3a Leg Press

T3b Hamstring Curl

T3c Quadriceps Extension

T3d Calf Raise

	Target Rep Range	Weight	Target Effort	# of Sets
Week 1	15 to 20	?	E	3 to 4
Week 2	15 to 20	?	M	3 to 4
Week 3	15 to 20	?	H	1 to 2
Week 4	12 to 15	?	E	3 to 4
Week 5	12 to 15	?	M	3 to 4
Week 6	12 to 15	?	H	1 to 2
Week 7	10 to 12	?	E	3 to 4
Week 8	10 to 12	?	M	3 to 4
Week 9	10 to 12	?	H	1 to 2
Week 10	8 to 10	?	E	3 to 4
Week 11	8 to 10	?	M	3 to 4
Week 12	8 to 10	?	H	1 to 2

Steel Helm

Steel Helm is an intensification progression based on the basic Wave LP; it can reasonably follow any such progression. Consider Steel Helm after cycles of Riptide, Undertow, Iron Tides, or Abyssal Wake.

T1 Maximal Strength

Continue adding weight to the RM set in Week 12, skipping the singles after. For example, if you set a 3RM at 225 pounds, work up to a new 3RM at 230 pounds in Week 13. Continue this intensification progression of adding weight each week until you hit a new 1RM. It should take about three weeks of gradual weight progression (intensification) to go from a hard 3RM (or more) to a hard 1RM.

The length of Steel Helm will vary depending on what program it continues from. For example, if running an accumulation cycle of GG Wave LP, the RM will be higher. Steel Helm is an intensification cycle that leads to a 1RM attempt in the final week (however long that might be). Conversely, if following Riptide with Steel Helm, the RM's are heavier, so you'll find a 1RM sooner.

T2 Strength Endurance

Find a 5RM at an easy target effort. (For example, picking up after pushing your old 5RM at the end of Abyssal Wake). This way, you can perform triples on its VDS. Next week, add weight, aiming to hold the same 5RM at a moderate effort. Try maintaining the same VDS, but reduce the reps per set from triples to doubles if needed. Next week, add weight again, aiming to maintain a 5RM with a hard effort.

Perform 4 to 6 doubles if possible, or singles if needed. This is a three-week progression of intensification, moving from the T2 side of the "bridge weight" 5RM to the T1 side.

Repeat this progression every three weeks, progressing from an easy 5RM followed by triples to a hard 5RM followed by singles, adding weight each week.

T3 Hypertrophy

Cycle through the T3 and T2 bridge reps range, going from 10 to 12 reps in week 1 at a moderate effort, to 8 to 10 in week 2, also at a moderate effort. Then, in the 3rd week, repeat the same weights as in week 2, aiming to make those now hard-effort sets in the higher-rep range (around 12 reps per set, if possible).

Wave Breaker

A progression biased towards strength rather than hypertrophy. Wave Breaker was formerly published as Ultra High Frequency Undulating Progression on my blog… a mouthful. My favorite period of Wave Breaker was when I trained only the squat and press as T1 and T2, which is why I used that example.

Base your own training plan on this progression model. You may prefer a split schedule, which is fine. Examples follow. Wave Breaker does not have a weekly progression like the previous example programs. This is because it requires much more auto-regulation. Adding weight to an RM when you are able, after you've hit volume targets for each respective day.

Examples: *Shift these volume targets to your goals.*

Session A: Once a weight has been pushed to a limit of 10 singles or a 5RM, add weight.

Session B: Once a 5RM weight is successfully pushed to a 6RM, add weight—no need to apply the full VDS amount before adding weight, as shown in the example.

Session C: Same progression as above, but starting at an 8RM and pushing to a 10RM. You may also use a heavier Session C than the example; do this by starting with a 6RM and pushing to an 8RM. If you choose a heavier session C, your work capacity in the T2 should be robust, so a full extension of T2 VDS is unlikely to leave you exhausted for the next session.

Though I run this as a full-body rotation across the three sessions, it can also be a body part or upper/lower split if you prefer. Examples are provided further down.

Note: Front and lateral delts, pecs, and triceps get significant work without specific T3s when pressing and/or benching several times per week. Add those only if you feel they are explicitly needed in your T3 schedule. This is why most of the T3s below are back, abs, biceps, and legs. But as always, you should adapt this to your individual needs and goals.

Incorporate rest days according to your schedule and recovery ability.

General Gainz - Wave Breaker

A rotating three-day progression.   Example Workout.
Best for improving lifts via skill development.
A repeated workout (same volume and weight for an
exercise) defaults to density progression.
Day 1 [A]: Heavy (Weight) Hard (Effort).
Day 2 [B]: Medium (Weight) Moderate (Effort).
Day 3 [C]: Light (Weight) Easy (Effort).

Session A

(T1) Heavy Range
Hard Effort
T1 Upper & Lower
Ex: Press & Squat
Singles only or 1-3RM attempt

Progress singles up to five total before attempting to add
weight or attempting an RM on the last single to
determine progression for the next workout; either add
weight or do more singles or attempt a RM.

Up to 10 singles or a 5RM can be performed on this day,
building volume while limiting rest before adding weight
or attempting a new heavy RM.
T3: Abs

Session B

(T2) Moderate Range
Moderate Effort
T2 Upper & Lower
Ex: Press & Squat
5RM & 6RM (Bridge Weights)

5RM to a 6RM; "bridge weights" in General Gainz.
Follow RM sets with half-sets of 2 to 3 reps per set.

Progress a 5RM to a 6RM+3x6 before adding weight via
push & extend actions. Complete a minimum of 3 to 4
sets after the RM with a goal of 6 half-sets before
increasing the RM weight.
T3: Back

Session C

(T2) Light Range
Easy Effort
T2 Upper & Lower
Ex: Press & Squat
8RM & 10RM

8RM to 10RM with half-sets after. Followed up with half-
sets of 4 to 6 reps per set.

Progress from an 8RM to a 10RM+5x6 before adding
weight. Complete 3 to 4 VDS after the RM with a
minimum goal of 6 half-sets before increasing the RM
weight. Three-quarter VDS can be used. If so, only 4
VDS may be necessary before a successful RM push.
T3: Biceps

Wave Breaker – Example Splits

Two Days (Full Body)

General Gainz - Wave Beaker 2 Day Full Body

Workout #1

T1	**Bench**	A (Heavy)
T2	**Deadlift** (or Variation)	B (Moderate)
T2	**Squat** (or Variation)	C (Light)
T3	**Back & Abs**	

Workout #2

T1	**Squat**	A (Heavy)
T2	**Press** (or Variation)	B (Moderate)
T2	**Bench** (or Variation)	C (Light)
T3	**Biceps & Legs**	

With this schedule, rotate your exercises through the [A/B/C] progression every 3 weeks.

Three Days (Full Body)

General Gainz - Wave Breaker 3 Day Full Body

Workout #1

T1	**Squat**	A (Heavy)
T2	**Bench** (or Variation)	B (Moderate)
T2	**Deadlift** (or Variation)	C (Light)
T3	**Back**	

Workout #2

T1	**Bench**	A (Heavy)
T2	**Deadlift** (or Variation)	B (Moderate)
T2	**Squat** (or Variation)	C (Light)
T3	**Abs**	

Workout #3

T1	**Deadlift**	A (Heavy)
T2	**Squat** (or Variation)	B (Moderate)
T2	**Bench** (or Variation)	C (Light)
T3	**Legs & Biceps**	

This is a powerlifting-biased schedule. Rotate through pressing, cleans, and other suitable exercises across the tiers as desired.

Four Days (Full Body)

General Gainz - Wave Breaker 4 Day Full Body

Workout #1

T1	**Squat**	A (Heavy)
T2	**Bench** (or Variation)	B (Moderate)
T2	**Deadlift** (or Variation)	C (Light)
T3	**Abs**	

Workout #2

T1	**Bench**	A (Heavy)
T2	**Deadlift** (or Variation)	B (Moderate)
T2	**Press** (or Variation)	C (Light)
T3	**Back & Biceps**	

Workout #3

T1	**Deadlift**	A (Heavy)
T2	**Press** (or Variation)	B (Moderate)
T2	**Bench** (or Variation)	C (Light)
T3	**Legs**	

Workout #4

T1	**Press**	A (Heavy)
T2	**Squat** (or Variation)	B (Moderate)
T2	**Row** (or Variation)	C (Light)
T3	**Chest & Shoulders**	

This schedule requires no tier rotation. However, rotating variations within workouts is suggested.

Four Days (Split)

General Gainz - Wave Breaker 4
Day Split

Workout #1

T1	**Squat**	A (Heavy)
T2	**Squat** (or Variation)	B (Moderate)
T2	**Deadlift** (or Variation)	C (Light)
T3	**Legs**	

Workout #2

T1	**Bench**	A (Heavy)
T2	**Bench** (or Variation)	B (Moderate)
T2	**Press** (or Variation)	C (Light)
T3	**Chest & Shoulders**	

Workout #3

T1	**Deadlift**	A (Heavy)
T2	**Deadlift** (or Variation)	B (Moderate)
T2	**Squat** (or Variation)	C (Light)
T3	**Back & Abs**	

Workout #4

T1	**Press**	A (Heavy)
T2	**Press** (or Variation)	B (Moderate)
T2	**Bench** (or Variation)	C (Light)
T3	**Arms**	

This schedule requires no tier rotation. Keeping T1 and T2 the same in a single workout makes the session faster because you don't have to warm up for the T2 lift; just move straight to T2 after your T1 work. However, swapping variations is suggested for higher frequency. For example, putting the T2 bench with the T1 press and vice versa. Likewise for squat and deadlift. But such workouts can take a while in the gym.

Five Days (Split, Less Frequent Lift Rotation)

General Gainz - Wave Breaker 5 Day Split

Workout #1

T1 Squat — A (Heavy)

T2 Squat (or Variation) — B (Moderate)

T2 Deadlift (or Variation) — C (Light)

T3 Abs

Workout #2

T1 Bench — A (Heavy)

T2 Incline (or Variation) — B (Moderate)

T2 Press (or Variation) — C (Light)

T3 Shoulders & Biceps

Workout #3

T1 Deadlift — A (Heavy)

T2 Squat (or Variation) — B (Moderate)

T2 Lunge (or Variation) — C (Light)

T3 Legs

Workout #4

T1 Press — A (Heavy)

T2 Incline (or Variation) — B (Moderate)

T2 Bench (or Variation) — C (Light)

T3 Chest & Triceps

Workout #5

T1 Row — A (Heavy)

T2 Row (or Variation) — B (Moderate)

T2 Pull Up (or Variation) — C (Light)

T3 Back & Biceps

This schedule requires no tier rotation. However, rotating variations within workouts is recommended.

Six- and seven-day Wave Breaker schedules can be configured if desired. The examples above are sufficient to customize further this progression and its potential schedule to your needs.

Treasure Hunter

PR Every Day. This requires extreme flexibility and meticulous tracking of training data to achieve a higher success rate. While fun, it is demanding. I enjoy this approach after a heavier training period, before moving into a lighter one. This helps me more accurately identify my RM ability in T2, while also allowing time to build work capacity through VDS development in both T1 and T2. Plus, it's fun to PR curls, calf raises, and whatever other odd lifts that fit into your training plan.

Wave through exercises for more opportunities to PR, utilizing that data to identify exercises you will train in the following wave of more structured training.

Rule #1

The first lift of every session is a T1 RM PR attempt—any RM in the T1 range at any effort target. This does not have to be the same T1 RM each week.

If an RM attempt seems unreasonable, meaning an RM attempt at any weight or effort seems unwise due to fatigue, etc., attempt to beat the overall volume of last week's RM via singles at the same weight.

Example:

Week 1: 4RM@545(H) [PR]

Week 2: Skip RM@545(E/H) 1 x 6

Here, in the second week, when the weight is repeated, the RM is skipped (because it was the PR last week), so only the

VDS are completed at that weight. Effort ratings are applied to the first and last singles: Easy / Hard. The final single completed should be at the RM's effort rating from the week before, or easier.

If the RM PR was successful, do not follow up with any additional volume. If unsuccessful and energy and rep quality are still acceptable, perform singles with that weight to match or exceed the previous PR. Do not follow the RM with any singles if you suspect the quality of those reps will be unacceptable.

Rule #2

The second lift of the session follows the same logic, but for the T2. You may perform up to three T2 exercises in a Treasure Hunter-inspired workout.

A. If you perform one T2 exercise in the workout, either the RM must be a PR or the total volume completed via VDS (if the RM was skipped).
B. If you perform two T2 exercises in one workout, the first must be an RM PR attempt. Whether it is successful or not, do not follow the first exercise's RM with half-sets; skip that additional work and move directly to the second T2 exercise in the workout. With this exercise, perform only the volume sets from a recent T2 RM PR. The goal of this second T2 is to PR the total volume of the VDS (push half-sets to three-quarters and/or extend the half-sets).
C. If you perform three T2 exercises in the workout, the first two are PR attempts only. No additional VDS after these RM sets with these first two exercises. The third exercise is a VDS total volume PR attempt.

D. Cycle the T2 exercises weekly, alternating which ones are RM PR attempts only and which ones are VDS total volume PRs.

Rule #3

Complete three to four T3 exercises in the workout, depending on your work capacity. Perform one set with the first one or two exercises, setting a PR in the 8RM to 15RM range with no further sets.

For the remaining exercises, PR the total volume (with associated effort targets), following the same logic as above.

Rule #4

Rotating lifts every session makes it easier to find PRs.

For example, you may rotate through vertical pushes for T1 (standard barbell, specialty bars, dumbbells, kettlebells, log, sandbag, etc.), then hit horizontal pulls (row variations) for T2, wrapping up the session with a variety of upper-body lifts for the T3s. This would make an "upper body" Treasure Hunter workout. You may prefer a different kind of split, whether by lift or full body, depending on your schedule.

Treasure Hunter was born out of a game I developed in the early days of General Gainz. I would use this to help me build a workout on days that would otherwise be rest days. Or during weeks when I hadn't ironed out my next program. At first, I just did it with T3s. But that soon turned into using it for T2s and T1s.

Sea-Wolf

Much like Treasure Hunter, Sea-Wolf is a training plan that heavily emphasizes the importance of the RM sets. Sea-Wolf fully excludes the VDS, whether T1 or T2, and limits T3 to a single set. Because of this, the RM should be pushed to at least a moderate effort, if not a hard effort. While hitting PRs each session is a plus, it is not necessary when running Sea-Wolf. The goal is to work up to a single set, then move onto the next exercise, and the next, and the next…

Because of this, I've had the most success with this training format when using upper/lower, push/pull/legs, or body-part splits. This reduces the need to warm up for a completely new lift, such as going from bench press to deadlift.

Sea-Wolf is a great training plan for those who value variety and those who need quick workouts. These sessions are fun and move fast. While I haven't hit many PRs on T1 and T2 lifts while using the Sea-Wolf format, it has allowed me to PR on many T3 exercises. This is because far less training volume is done in the T1 and T2, so more hard effort can be applied in the T3. For this reason, it is a great plan to move some T3 exercises into the T2 (for better development later), or vice versa, which is why it operates in the Bridge Weight ranges (T1's crossing into T2's, and T3's the same).

What I find most fun about Sea-Wolf is completing the workout against the clock, trying to get as many different exercises done within the time I've set. That might be 20 minutes on a busy day or 60 on an average day. This could result in 6 different RM sets completed and perhaps up to 20. For each lift, a few warm-up sets could be completed, but as I go through the workout, fewer warm-ups are needed, and by the end, none; I'll just take the curl bar with the weight I want and go for my hard-effort RM set, for example.

Generally, Sea-Wolf is an adventurous, demanding training plan that affords opportunities to progress that are less emphasized in the previously described concepts. That said, it is easy to go overboard, so be mindful of your ability and recovery capacity.

Below are a few examples; you can, of course, have more or fewer exercises.

Sea-Wolf Push/Pull/Legs Example

General Gainz Sea-Wolf P/P/L
Example Push Workout

Tier	Exercise	RM
T1	Press	3 to 5
T1b	Incline Bench	3 to 5
T2a	Close Grip Bench	6 to 10
T2b	Dips	6 to 10
T3a	Pec Fly	8 to 12
T3b	Triceps Push Down	8 to 12
T3c	Overhead Triceps Extension	10 to 15
T3d	Lateral Delt Raise	10 to 15

Example Pull Workout

Tier	Exercise	RM
T1	Weighted Pull-Ups	3 to 5
T1b	Barbell Row	3 to 5
T2a	Underhand Pull Down	6 to 10
T2b	Shrugs	6 to 10
T3a	Barbell Pull Overs	8 to 12
T3b	Cable Upright Row	8 to 12
T3c	Preacher Curls	10 to 15
T3d	Rear Delt Fly	10 to 15

Example Legs Workout

Tier	Exercise	RM
T1	Squat	3 to 5
T1b	Front Squat	3 to 5
T2a	Romanian Deadlift	6 to 10
T2b	Leg Press	6 to 10
T3a	Leg Curls	8 to 12
T3b	Leg Extensions	8 to 12
T3c	Calf Raise	10 to 15
T3d	Kickbacks	10 to 15

Sea-Wolf Upper/Lower Example

General Gainz Sea-Wolf Upper/Lower
Example Upper Workout A

Tier	Exercise	RM
T1a	Press	3 to 5
T1b	Lat Pull Down	3 to 5
T2a	Bench	6 to 10
T2b	Bent Over Row	6 to 10
T3a	Overhead Triceps Extension	8 to 12
T3b	Preacher Curl	8 to 12
T3c	Pec Fly	10 to 15
T3d	Rear Delt Fly	10 to 15

Example Lower Workout A

Tier	Exercise	RM
T1a	Squat	3 to 5
T1b	Power Clean	3 to 5
T2a	Leg Press	6 to 10
T2b	Calf Raise	6 to 10
T3a	Leg Extensions	8 to 12
T3b	Leg Curls	8 to 12
T3c	Hip Abduction	10 to 15
T3d	Hip Adduction	10 to 15

Example Upper Workout B

Tier	Exercise	RM
T1a	Bench	3 to 5
T1b	Bent Over Row	3 to 5
T2a	Incline Bench	6 to 10
T2b	Underhand Lat Pull Down	6 to 10
T3a	Dips	8 to 12
T3b	Face Pull	8 to 12
T3c	Barbell Pull Over	10 to 15
T3d	Shrugs	10 to 15

Example Lower + Abs Workout B

Tier	Exercise	RM
T1a	Deadlift	3 to 5
T1b	Front Squat	3 to 5
T2a	Lunges	6 to 10
T2b	Romanian Deadlift	6 to 10
T3a	Decline Sit-Ups	8 to 12
T3b	Ab Straps	8 to 12
T3c	Pallof Press	10 to 15
T3d	High/Low Woodchopper	10 to 15

Sea-Wolf Full-Body

General Gainz Sea-Wolf Full-Body
Example Full-Body Workout A

Tier	Exercise	RM
T1a	Squat	3 to 5
T2a	Cleans	6 to 10
T3a	Bulgarian Split Squat	8 to 12
T3b	Leg Curls	10 to 15
T3c	Leg Extensions	10 to 15
T1b	Press	3 to 5
T2b	Underhand Lat Pull Down	6 to 10
T3d	Incline Bench	8 to 12
T3e	Row	10 to 15
T3f	Lateral Delt Raise	10 to 15

Example Full-Body Workout B

Tier	Exercise	RM
T1a	Bench	3 to 5
T2a	Row	6 to 10
T3a	Dips	8 to 12
T3b	Pull-Ups	10 to 15
T3c	Rear Delt Fly	10 to 15
T1b	Deadlift	3 to 5
T2b	Front Squat	6 to 10
T3d	Calf Raise	8 to 12
T3e	DB Side Crunch	10 to 15
T3f	Decline Sit-Ups	10 to 15

Dice Gainz

Sometimes we have limited time to train, or we're between pre-planned progressions, yet still want to train. Dice Gainz removes much of the thinking, allowing you to lift and enjoy training.

For those who struggle with analysis paralysis, Dice Gainz may be a welcome remedy. Give yourself up to chance (but with some sensible rules in place to guide you).

T1 Maximal Strength (First Roll)

- Use a single d6 (six-sided die).

- The number rolled determines the Rep Max (RM) attempt
  (e.g., roll a 4 → find a 4RM).

- Follow with an equal number of singles at the same weight (4RM → 4 additional singles). As usual with GG, singles may be extended by up to 3 beyond the RM value (4RM → 7 additional singles; 6RM → 9 additional singles) based on effort.

T2 Strength Endurance (Second Roll)

- Use a single d6.

- Roll +5 determines RM target
  (e.g., roll a 3 → find an 8RM).

- Follow with half-sets. If the RM is an odd number and at hard effort (meaning zero reps in reserve), round down these half-sets. 7RM → VDS are three reps per set. Perform 4 to 6 half-sets after the RM set, based on effort.

- Option: Add a second T2 exercise to a workout (roll for this one separately or use the same RM value for the second exercise). Up to two T2 exercises are allowed in a workout based on the lifter's skill, work capacity, and recovery.

T3 Hypertrophy (Third Roll)

- Roll a single d6.

- Roll +10 determines RM target (e.g., roll a 5 → find a 15RM).

- Perform two more sets with the same weight, trying to match the reps of the first set.

- Perform up to four different T3 exercises per workout.

Additional Rules for Playability

1. Exercise Selection (How to Pick Lifts)

Instead of random selection for exercises, a structured pool of exercises can be used:

- **Pre-Select Options**: The lifter can assign a set of exercises for each tier before rolling, knowing already what lifts they will be doing before they roll. In this case, the first roll is for the chosen T1 lift, the second roll for the chosen T2 lift, and the following rolls for the chosen T3 lifts.

- **Dice-Assigned Selection**: If randomness is desired, assign a number to each exercise and roll to determine which lift to perform for the RM that was the result of the first roll.

Example for a d6 roll on T1 (compound lifts):

1 = Squat
2 = Deadlift
3 = Bench
4 = Overhead Press
5 = Front Squat
6 = Deficit Deadlift

For example:

First Roll: Die lands on a 3, meaning you'll perform a 3RM.

Second Roll: Die lands on a 4, meaning you'll do that 3RM with the Overhead Press.

The same could be applied to T2 (secondary lifts) and T3 (accessory movements) during a workout.

2. Overriding Rolls (Fatigue & Readiness Rule)

- If an absurdly difficult RM comes up (example: rolling a 1 for T1 and having to attempt a 1RM cold), allow one override roll per session, but the second roll must be accepted.

    o   In this case, if feeling fatigued, roll again for:

- 1-3 → Keep the original roll.

    - 4-6 → Adjust by ±1 rep to fit energy levels.

- Alternatively, keep whatever RM sets you want to avoid out of consideration. Roll a 1RM or 2RM and don't want to? Roll until you get the RM you want. But don't be mad if the dice *really* want you to do that 1RM.

3. Weighted Dice Rule (Progressive Overload: Intensification or Accumulation)

- If the lifter completes a full workout using a rolled RM, they may use a weighted dice rule next time:

    - Instead of rolling, repeat that workout but heavier (intensification), or you can repeat the workout with the same weight but do more reps (accumulation). With accumulation, you can try pushing the weight to a higher RM or adding reps to the VDS.

    - The dice determined the workout last time. You determine how to progress this time, whether by adding weight or by increasing reps at the same weight as in the last workout.

4. Failure Rule

- If a lifter fails their RM set (can't complete reps):

- o **Move immediately to the VDS, extending beyond the completed RM if quality permits** (singles if T1, half-sets if T2): For example, if a 5RM was targeted but a 3RM at a hard effort was performed because the estimated weight was too heavy, do singles according to the 3RM guidelines, not the 5RM. Meaning, up to six singles after the 3RM.

- o **Alternate rule:** Convert failed reps into singles, but do not go beyond the rolled for RM value. Meaning, if you only get 3 reps on a rolled 5RM, finish two additional singles, then move to the T2 exercise. This would be the better choice if you're fatigued and the rep quality is subpar.

- o On T2s, **limit half-sets to 3 or 4**, based on rep quality and fatigue after a failed T2 RM attempt. There's no need to extend sets when the RM itself was missed because the effort, weight, and quality were subpar. (Ex: Only doing a 6RM when an 8RM was the target.)

5. Chaos Multiplier (Advanced Play: Intensification or Accumulation)

- Introduce a separate roll for extra difficulty or variety:

  - o **Odd number roll (1, 3, 5) → Push or Extend VDS to their limits,** whether the T1 or T2. Example: if an 8RM was performed, the half-sets might be pushed to 5's (instead of 4's), making for a three-quarter set progression. Or, six VDS must be completed.

- o **Even number roll (2, 4, 6)** → Increase intensity by **adding weight to the VDS after the RM.** Example: if a 5RM was performed at 225 pounds, perform the follow-up singles at 230 pounds.

Additional Layers for Dice Gainz

Now that the core structure and some options are defined, the following deload mechanisms, challenge modes, and long-term progress-tracking options are introduced to round out the system.

1. Deload Mechanisms (Auto-Regulation & Periodization)

To prevent burnout, lifters should occasionally back off from highly demanding sessions for a few days. Dice Gainz can incorporate deloading in two ways:

A. Automatic Deload Rolls

- Every 4th or 5th session, roll a d6 before the workout:

    - o **1-3 → Full Workout** (Normal rules apply).

    - o **4-5 → Reduce Volume** (Cut RM VDS in half).

    - o **6 → Reduce Intensity & Volume** (aim for easy RM's and reduced VDS).

B. Controlled Deload

- Instead of rolling for deloads, lifters can pre-schedule every 4th or 5th session as a deload:

    o **T1:** Roll for RM but reduce weight by aiming for easy efforts.

    o **T1 & T2:** Keep RM targets but reduce VDS.

    o **T3** keep all sets at easy effort targets and/or perform fewer than usual.

C. Deload by Performance

- If the same RM roll fails twice in a row, the lifter must deload the next session.

2. Challenge Modes (Game Variations)

These add variety for lifters looking to spice things up.

A. "Push Your Luck" Mode

- After completing an RM set, roll a d6:

    o **1-2 → Increase weight** for VDS.

    o **3-4 → Normal rules apply.**

    o **5-6 → Extend VDS required** (+3 extra singles beyond T1 RM, 6 half-sets for T2).

B. "Death Roll" Mode (Max Fatigue Challenge)

- After finishing all exercises, roll a d6:

    o **Odd number:** Choose any one completed exercise and perform one final RM set.

o   The lift can be decided by the lifter (to limit risk exposure) or decided by the dice with a subsequent roll (if the lifter's readiness allows).

o   **Even number:** No extra work.

C. "Double or Nothing" Mode (High-Stakes Risk-Reward)

- After a T1 RM attempt, roll a d6:

    o   **1-3 → No changes** (continue with normal singles).

    o   **4-6 → Must retry the RM at a heavier weight.**

D. "Dice Gauntlet" Mode (Volume Challenge)

- At the end of a workout, roll for:

    o   **1-2 → Workout ends.**

    o   **3-4 → Pick any T2 or T3 exercise and do one more RM set.**

    o   **6 → Pick any T2 or T3 exercise and perform the full RM + VDS or MRS.**

- You may roll for these or predetermine the RM value, weight, and effort targets.

Long-Term Progress Tracking

Since dice determine workouts, tracking progress ensures progression and prevents stagnation.

A. Logging System

- Each session, record:

    o **Rolled RM targets.**

    o **Actual reps achieved.**

    o **VDS/MRS performed.**

    o **Weight used for all sets.**

    o **Effort Rating (Easy 2+ RiR, Moderate 1RiR, Hard 0RiR)**

This helps identify trends (e.g., if 5RM rolls are getting easier, it's time to increase weight).

B. "Level-Up" System

- After a successful RM, the lifter may:

    o Keep that lift but use a heavier weight for all future rolls (progressive overload).

    o After several successful RMs with an exercise in a workout, swap out exercises to keep variety high.

C. Goal-Based Customization

- If the goal is strength, prioritize heavier RM rolls:

    o On a d6 roll for T1, lifters can re-roll 6s and 5s once per session.

- If the goal is hypertrophy, prioritize higher rep rolls:

    o On a d6 roll for T2 and T3 exercises, lifters can re-roll 6s and 5s once per session.

Expanding Dice Gainz: Endless Possibilities

Here are additional challenges, multiplayer rules, and sport-specific adaptations to make Dice Gainz a truly dynamic training system.

1. Additional Challenges

For those who crave unpredictability, here are even more challenge modes.

A. "Sudden Death" Mode (Single Attempt Maxing)

- Roll a d6 at the start of a session:

    - **1** → Attempt a 1RM (T1) at a hard effort, aiming for a PR.

    - **2** → Attempt a 10RM (T2) at a hard effort, aiming for a PR.

    - **3** → No change, train as usual.

    - **4** → Instead of singles after a T1 or half-sets after a T2, perform two RM sets with the same weight. Ex: a 4RM@225 followed by a 2 or 3RM @225.

    - **5** → All T3 sets are to failure.

    - **6** → Choose your own challenge (repeat last week's most difficult set, or attempt a PR, etc.).

B. "Dense Wave" Mode (Density Challenge)

- Roll for T1, T2, and T3 as usual.

- Then roll for rest:

    - **1-3** → Rest 10 seconds less for T1, 20 less for T2, and 30 less for T3.

    - **4-6** → Rest 20 seconds less for T1, 30 less for T2, and 40 less for T3.

C. "Break the Chain" Mode (Fatigue Mastery)

- Each time you fail a rep on an RM attempt, roll a d6:

    - **1-3** → Move on with VDS as previously detailed.

    - **4-6** → Try the RM again, but lighter. Then keep the VDS at the original heavier weight, which the first RM attempt failed at.

D. "Survivor" Mode

- Set a time limit for the workout.

- Roll for T1, T2, and T3 as usual, but only one set is performed per exercise.

- Move through one T1, one to three T2s, and as many T3 exercises as possible in the remaining time, or until all T3s assigned to numbers of the die are completed.

- Roll for each exercise (either at random or preselected from a list) and each RM.

- Limit rest to the best of your ability.

D. "Hero's Journey" Mode (RPG-Leveling System)

This is just the beginning of what could be a long game of lifting weights and getting stronger. Some lifters benefit from gamification. Dice Gainz is excellent for those motivated by such goals and offers a unique approach to training progression.

Lifters can "level up" their Dice Gainz experience:

- **Earn XP** by:

    o **Adding weight** to RM sets → +1 Strength.

    o **Adding rep**s to the same weight → +1 Endurance.

    o **Completing all T3s** in 10 consecutive workouts → +1 Size.

    o **Hitting a PR** while following the dice → +1 Power.

    o **Streaking 10 workouts** without an unplanned day off → +1 Wisdom.

- **XP unlocks perks** like:

    o One free reroll per session.

    o Bonus multiplier rolls (adding exercises to workouts if you streak your T3s.)

    o Ability to choose an exercise once per session instead of rolling.

Determine your perk thresholds based on your experience level. Don't put these too far out of reach when starting out.

2. Multiplayer Rules

If training with a partner or group, these rules make Dice Gainz competitive.

A. "Head-to-Head" Mode

- **Two lifters** roll for T1, T2, and T3 exercises, using the same target RMs

- Whoever completes a personal record on their RM set wins that tier.

- If an RM is not PR'd, whoever completes the most total reps across all VDS wins.

    - Lifters can push and/or extend VDS after the RM to the best of their ability to beat the opponent.

- Losing lifter must do a penalty round of one additional VDS for that tier.

B. "Draft Mode"

- Each lifter rolls all three tiers in advance.

- They can trade one RM value with another player before lifting starts.

- Adds strategy: Do you take the easier roll or give yourself a harder challenge?

C. "Dice King" Challenge

- Over a 4-week cycle, players keep score:

    - +1 point for completing RM rolls as prescribed.

- o +2 points for setting a PR on a rolled RM.

  - o +2 points for setting a PR on VDS.

  - o -1 point for failing an RM.

  - o -1 point for losing the PR's (either RM or VDS).

- At the end, the highest score wins. The winner assigns an extra T3 exercise for the loser in the next cycle. (Pick a T3 that's going to benefit your lifting partner.)

3. Sport-Specific Adaptations

Dice Gainz can be customized for powerlifting, weightlifting, CrossFit, and strongman.

A. Powerlifting Version

- **T1:** Main competition lift: Squat (1,4), Bench (2,5), or Deadlift (3,6).

- **T2:** Variation: Paused Squats (1,4), Close-Grip Bench (2,5), Romanian Deadlifts (3,6).

- **T3:** Accessory work (Rows, Core, Unilateral Work). Assigned lifts to support T1s.

- **Rule Additions:**

  - o If a 1-2 is rolled on T1, lifter must perform a paused variation.

  - o If a 5 or 6 is rolled on a T1 or T2, use the weight from the most recent RM, perform the VDS only, pausing that weight if possible.

B. Olympic Weightlifting Version

- **T1:** Snatch (1,3,5) and Clean & Jerk (2,4,6).

- **T2:** Pull or Squat variation: Squat (1), Front Squat (2), Snatch Pull (3), Clean Pull (4), Romanian Deadlift (5), Muscle Clean or Muscle Snatch (6; lifter's choice).

- **T3:** Squats & Assistance (Overhead Squat, pull-ups, etc.). Assigned to support T1 lifts.

- **Rule Additions:**

  - If a 1 is rolled on T1, the lifter must go for a heavy single.

  - If a 4 to 6 is rolled on a T1, the lifter must go for singles of equivalent value instead of the RM. Singles should be at a weight estimated to be the RM. For example, doing four singles instead of a 4RM, but using the 4RM weight (or an estimated value).

  - If a 4 to 6 is rolled on T2, the lifter must perform extra paused reps at their most challenging position (pause squats, overhead holds, etc.).

C. CrossFit Version

- **T1:** Strength-based barbell movement (Squat, Deadlift, Press).

- **T2:** Metcon-focused movement (Kettlebell Swings, Thrusters, DB Snatches).

- **T3:** Bodyweight/gymnastics or conditioning (Pull-ups, Burpees, Rowing).

- Rule Additions:

  - If an odd number is rolled on T2, perform EMOM-style.

  - If an even number is rolled on a T2, perform sets with minimal rest.

  - If a 6 is rolled on T3, add a 400m run between sets.

D. Strongman Version

- **T1:** Max Effort Movement (Log Press, Axle Deadlift, Yoke Carry).

- **T2:** Repetition Movement (Tire Flips, Keg Loads, Farmers Carries).

- **T3:** Grip/Core/Cardio Component (Sandbag Carries, Weighted Planks, Hill Sprints).

- Rule Additions:

  - If a 1 or 2 is rolled on T1, do an extra-long hold at the top of the lift.

  - If a 6 is rolled on a T1, do two RM sets with that exercise, totaling six reps.

  - If a 6 is rolled on a T2, perform a 20RM instead.

  - If a 1 is rolled on T3, add a finisher (sled drag, heavy carry for distance).

4. Advanced Progression Systems

These ensure long-term growth while keeping Dice Gainz unpredictable.

A. "Cycle Progression" Mode

- Every 3 weeks, lifters fix their workouts from the previous 3 weeks, adding weight to the same lifts and same volume.

B. "Bias Rolls" for Specialization

- If a lifter has a weak point (e.g., pressing strength), they can roll twice for T1 and pick the higher number to push that weakness.

C. "Legacy Rolls" for Strength Cycles

- If a lifter completes a full workout cycle at a given RM and it comes up in the next workout again, go for the next heaviest RM instead.

    o Example: If 4RM was successful last workout and comes up again this workout, instead of repeating the 4RM but heavier, go even heavier and aim for a 3RM.

Epilogue: Physicality, Creativity, Consciousness

Introduction

What follows is an explanation of why I lift. However, these concepts can be applied more broadly beyond lifting and physical fitness. While these reflections do not underlie General Gainz, it was while training within that framework that I discovered my reason for training. I hope you, the reader, find this perspective helpful to your fitness endeavors and to everything else in your life, as it has been in mine.

The Road to Nowhere

Why do you lift?
Is it cathartic?
Relaxing?
An outlet for something?
Or is it a journey?
A road
to a place
with a number that's pleasing?
If your rage never fades,
is your therapy working?
When your road is blocked,
will you stop walking?
No, you will not.
Why do you lift?
Is it the sound of the plates
And the smell of chalk in the air?
Or the commitment,
and effort,
and drive,
to realize yourself

on this road to nowhere?
Your hate cannot fuel this drive.
And the passion will turn to fog.
This road is long.
Its slope is steep.
What inside drives you on this Sisyphean feat?
If not anger, passion, or a number,
Why do you lift?
On this road to nowhere?

I wrote that poem nine years ago. At the time, I didn't have an answer to my question *why do you lift?* After working out every day for four years, I found one.

A Strange Loop

Philosopher and mathematician Douglas Hofstadter developed the concept of "strange loops" to explain how self-referential systems can create complex patterns and structures. His book "Gödel, Escher, Bach: An Eternal Golden Braid" describes the paradoxical, self-referential nature of certain systems. According to Hofstadter, a strange loop is a system that contains a self-referential structure which, when observed at a higher level of abstraction, creates a paradoxical situation. Hofstadter suggests that our lives are analogous to such paradoxical, strange loops.

In the case of physicality, creativity, and consciousness, the strange loop occurs when each of these elements refers to the other two, forming a feedback loop of increasing complexity. For example, physicality refers to how the body and the surrounding environment affect consciousness and creative output. Our consciousness influences how we experience physicality as our creative impulses shape both our physical actions and mental states. Creativity generates new ideas and expressions, but our physicality and consciousness also influence creativity. Our physical abilities and limitations shape how we express ourselves creatively, and our conscious experiences inform the content and style of our creative output. All the while, consciousness depends on our subjective experience of the world, grounded in our physical experiences, creative expressions, and understanding within it.

Our senses and actions shape how we perceive the world, fostering imaginative endeavors and deepening our understanding of it. Together, these three elements create a feedback loop of increasing complexity, with each one influencing and being influenced by the other two. This creates a strange loop that can generate endless patterns and structures, as well as new insights into the nature of our physicality, creativity, and consciousness.

Creativity is inherently physical. Some paint. Others dance. Life is in each. Action is observed in the brush strokes of the painter. Emotion is observed in the steps of the dancer. Action recorded in paint makes a lifeless canvas come to life. A dancer's flowing limbs make the theater another world. Both artists create and inspire, breathing life into space, their audiences, and themselves. Our physicality propels us through the strange loop that is us; our consciousness improves through creativity, requiring physicality.

As with traditional forms of artistic expression, a person lifting weights is creating. Individual compositions are merely slivers of the grand creation: the artist themselves within a single workout and the lifter, a product of many workouts. Regarding the lifter, they are simultaneously developing a sculpture of flesh while carefully practicing a choreography of exercises, for creations (actions) reflect the actor (creator). What is created is a mirror through which feedback is experienced and processed. Feedback provides direction; without it, progression is impossible. Without progression, through some creative act, we become mired and lost. Then our mind, spirit, and body become increasingly disconnected, until such detachment brings death to each part of us. The last of which, the body, when developed through creativity, retains and improves the former two. In this way, the triumvirate of self is governed. Our physicality receives feedback, in turn prompting more creativity from which our sense of self is developed.

The process of self-development is a loop that requires action to progress through. Creativity, being an act of physicality, whether singing, painting, lifting, etc., develops two mediums, the most important being the artist themselves. The inanimate comes alive through the actions of the creator. The canvas, the theatre, the piano, the barbell; each is dead before being acted upon. Through the creative process, the individual receives feedback that fosters self-awareness. The creator lives in their creations and the creations in their creator.

The strange loop arises when we consider that our physical bodies are not only passive tools of consciousness and creativity but are themselves products of conscious and creative processes. Our bodies change via self-reflection, self-awareness, and self-modification. Our physicality is intertwined in paradoxical self-reference. It is both the foundation and the product of our conscious and creative processes, which in turn shape and transform who we are. The interdependence of these three concepts creates a strange loop that is both hierarchical and heterarchical, sensible yet paradoxical, while highlighting the intricate and mysterious nature of the human experience.

Our physicality creates our consciousness, and our consciousness creates our physicality. We are what we do, and what we do, we become. When we stop doing, we stop being.

I lift, therefore I am.

As silly as it sounds, and as convoluted as that last section seems, the reality is that without consistent measures, we are incapable of observing the strange loop that is us. Our actions create a process. That process gives understanding, producing another action. Apart from this process, our reality, our very being, comes into question.

Cogito ergo sum. "I think, therefore I am," is the foundation on which René Descartes' philosophy of systematic doubt rests. Descartes, questioning his existence, found the question itself to be the answer. His philosophy is considered the origin of the modern scientific method. Then came Kurt Gödel's incompleteness theorems, published nearly 300 years later, proving self-reference is inherent in all complex logical systems; upon which Hofstadter theorizes strange loops, structures I argue give rise to consciousness out of a complex self-referential system, intrinsically tied to our physicality. As creative beings, we are the question and the answer within an internal and external experiment: ourselves and our world.

Can we honestly observe ourselves without generating feedback through the creative process? No. Therefore, one must find means to create consistent feedback. Doing so requires physicality. For me, that is lifting weights. And though it is a far simpler act than, say, playing an instrument, it is nevertheless a creative means that I have braided into my consciousness through consistent effort. Lifting is both quantifiable and qualitative, developmental, and sustainable. Therefore, it is and builds the structure through which my life flows.

Do not interpret this as an argument for being one-dimensional. I know who I am because of what I do, and I do what I know because that is who I am. And because I know who I am and what I can do, I am even more capable of doing things I do not know. We grow in capacity as we grow physically, and as we grow physically, we grow cognitively; these produce more creativity, and our first creation, incomplete until extinguished, is who we are.

Physicality, and more specifically the focus on improving my size, strength, and stamina, has allowed me to do more things than lift weights. Physical training is merely the process from which opportunity arises before me. Because I am fit, I am more capable. And because I am more capable, I can participate more in this strange thing we call life. The same can be true for you. Though it may seem daunting at first, know that the relationship between physicality, creativity, and consciousness is both the structure and the means of developing structure: You.

On a whim, I can climb a mountain or learn a new activity. When a blizzard hits, I can chop wood for hours and shovel snow that much longer. I can help myself, my family, and my neighbors because of the capacity I have developed through physical training. I am not special. This is the nature of our environment and who we are within it. Those interactions with new places, environments, objects, and people contribute to a feedback loop that develops our consciousness and forms our being.

When I am separated from the process that is braided into my being, that process being physical training, the awareness of my ability diminishes, and who I am fades with it. This is true for all of you and for any activity. A writer who experiences prolonged writer's block ceases to be a writer. Likewise, a musician who stops playing, a painter who stops painting, and, for Descartes, a thinker who stops thinking, stops being. Absence from feedback is death. To receive feedback, we must be consistent, put forth effort, and remain patient; three traits that bolster the physicality, creativity, and consciousness relationship.

Effort, Consistency, Patience

Anything worthwhile requires three things: Effort, Consistency, and Patience. Without each of those, the process is limited. As one fades, the other two do as well, making the day-to-day increasingly unfulfilling. Dissatisfaction comes as our patience wanes, effort dwindles, and consistency vanishes. Without one of the three, the other two produce insufficient fruit. It is their sum that is foundational to any endeavor, and self-development is the most critical endeavor.

Because who we are is born out of what we do, if we hope to live fulfilled, then we must put forth the effort by which the feedback we desire is generated. That effort must be consistent, day in, day out; otherwise, the feedback decreases in both quantity and quality, and with it, our growth. Patience yields time from which nourishing feedback is harvested. We grow when fed. Both the cultivation of food and its consumption take time, the former far longer than the latter. This is why creative acts must be consistent, for the feedback they produce is short-lived. Let this analogy be an encouragement. For effort can be exhausting, consistency monotonous, and patience thin, yet when grafted together, those branches produce fruits from a tree that is your life.

When ripe, our labors are enjoyed. Not merely by us alone, but by all those who may find shelter and nourishment beside us; those who return feedback: encouragement and criticism, kindness and cruelty, love and hate. Expect negativity and recognize that, with patience, it is possible to process all feedback constructively, turning it into fuel for sustained effort. The choice is ours. Do not be discouraged; it is not the input that determines the outcome, because we are not simply machines. Sure, it takes more effort and patience to repurpose negative feedback into positive results, but those solutions build hardier systems, the strange loops of existence.

Building a Complete System

A complete system is a set of interacting, interdependent components that work together to achieve a specific goal or purpose. It involves all the necessary elements and resources required for effective operation. A complete system may include hardware, software, data, procedures, personnel, and other operational or organizational components necessary to fulfill its intended purpose. It is a cohesive, integrated whole composed of various parts that work together to achieve a specific outcome. What is your desired outcome, and how are you developing and sustaining the complete system necessary to realize that goal? –Trick question. Even if you have a system, it will always be incomplete. Be encouraged! Allow me to explain.

Both action and inaction precede receiving feedback, because you are subject to an environment (including other people), and what you receive reflects the quality and consistency of your efforts. Your system will never be complete, so you should not expect yourself to have every means of receiving everything. That should not be a barrier to action. Inherent incompleteness requires physicality because it takes work: effort, consistency, and patience. These develop what is lacking. These allow you to explore the unknown, adding to your innate and eternal incompleteness. Let them piece together something new from what is available, developing creativity, discovering new solutions, increasing capacity, increasing your incompleteness, yet somehow, paradoxically, making you more whole.

All too often, we let a missing piece stop us from acting. We allow seemingly massive obstacles to impede our progress. Because of these missing pieces and barriers, we end up permanently operating within a limited and fragile system, simply because its boundaries are known. This is unfortunate because it confines us to a narrow set of solutions, narrowing our outcomes. It is possible that what we think is missing is an assumption, or that the perceived obstacle is an illusion. Operating on false premises guarantees inaccurate feedback. If you had everything you needed, would you be consistent? Would you put forth effort? Would you remain patient? No, because progress is not the fruit of completeness, but rather incompleteness.

Desiring completeness fruits analysis paralysis. That is, inactivity, meaning passive destruction, not active creation; ourselves being the first victim, rotting, ruining those around us because of our misguided desire for self-fulfillment; an impossibility. Instead, seek an ever-expanding understanding of your own incompleteness, seeing it as room to roam and grow, through challenge and the inevitable failures and victories born of actions taken within the mysterious unknown that is within and outside us. Do so knowing that building a complete system is impossible and not the goal, ever-expanding incompleteness is. Not for its end state, an unreachable destination, but for the enduring effort, patience, and consistency that our reaching demands. The byproducts of our actions are the harvested fruits of a lifetime spent caring for an imperfect yet productive orchard: yourself.

To prevent the development of a system lacking integrity, we must act first. That is, put forth the physical effort to discover the true nature of the system we are developing. Whether we act or not, we cannot be separated from the system that is part of us. It does not pause. Life goes on. The choice not to act is passivity, ultimately weakening the system that is us. Therefore, it is consistent physicality that both produces and holds together our incompleteness. Anything found lacking is discovered through physicality: the creative means of expanding a functioning, incomplete system.

Conclusion

The monotony of an endless loop is inescapable. It is who we are, and though the experiences and fruits (physicality and creativity) may change, the system itself does not. It can only grow more incompletely. Therefore, as we apply effort with consistency and patience, it is better to see the inevitable monotony as a positive force of our own creation. As erosion shaped the Grand Canyon, so too does the monotony we endure shape us, revealing our greatness more each day. This process fosters self-awareness through patient endurance, in time building the strength of character achievable only by remaining active and conscious in our development.

How does one remain, not wither in the environment, and be ground into dust? Assess what you do every day and determine if the loop you are in is developing your physicality, and therefore your creativity and consciousness. If one is lacking, so are the other two. To live, create something, and in that process, someone: you. Not sure what to do or how to do it? Act. Do not wait for the perfect time or for the feeling of having all the information, skills, or tools needed to produce the best results in the shortest time, so-called "optimal" (the favorite word of those who tend to suffer from analysis paralysis and other disordered behavior most). Remember that the process is the goal. Separating ourselves from doing, for any reason, is how we passively accept lifeless existence. Physicality is creativity is consciousness.

Do not seek perfection. Desire the process itself, for that is our strange loop. Braid into yourself ever more complex capabilities and creations, using those to receive all feedback with gratitude, even the negative! It is our effort and creativity that can turn such feedback into positive outcomes. Should anything be found lacking, remain consistent and patient, working through potential solutions. In due course, an incomplete system will be received wholly, with effort, consistency, and patience eroding the unnecessary, revealing the grander self within.

"Why do you lift?" Asked the poem that began this post. Because it helps me know who I am.